PASTORAL AESTHETICS

PASTORAL AESTHETICS

A Theological Perspective on Principlist Bioethics

Nathan Carlin

OXFORD
UNIVERSITY PRESS

OXFORD
UNIVERSITY PRESS

Oxford University Press is a department of the University of Oxford. It furthers the University's objective of excellence in research, scholarship, and education by publishing worldwide. Oxford is a registered trade mark of Oxford University Press in the UK and certain other countries.

Published in the United States of America by Oxford University Press
198 Madison Avenue, New York, NY 10016, United States of America.

CIP data is on file at the Library of Congress
ISBN 978-0-19-027014-8

9 8 7 6 5 4 3 2 1

Printed by Sheridan Books, Inc., United States of America

For Keatan King

I have nothing to offer except a way of looking at things.

—ERIK ERIKSON

CONTENTS

LIST OF ILLUSTRATIONS

law, including all related and neighboring rights: Public Domain Mark 1.0. This work is in the public domain in the United States because it was published (or registered with the US Copyright Office) before January 1, 1923. The source of the photograph is http://www.vggallery.com/painting/by_period/arles.htm. 140

Revised portions of these articles appear in the text, reprinted with permission from Springer Nature via the Copyright Clearance Center: Nathan Carlin, "Bioethics and Pastoral Concern: Some Possible New Directions in Pastoral Theology," *Pastoral Psychology* 62, no. 2 (2013): 129–138; and Nathan Carlin, "A Psychoanalytic Reading of *A Monster Calls*: Biblical Congruencies and Theological Implications," *Pastoral Psychology* 66, no. 6 (2017): 759–777.

PREFACE

This book is an integration of various strands of my academic life. While it may seem conceptual and academic—and indeed it is—this book at its core is deeply autobiographical, for it includes many of my conversation partners from the last twenty years. It weaves together my graduate education in psychology of religion and pastoral theology as well as my professional location as a teacher of humanities and ethics in a medical school. It was, therefore, very meaningful for me to write this book.

During my undergraduate education, I became interested in psychology of religion via Jeffrey Kripal at Westminster College. Next I went to Princeton Theological Seminary to study pastoral theology with Donald Capps and Robert Dykstra. I continued these studies during my doctoral program at Rice University with William Parsons and Jeffrey Kripal, who moved from Westminster to Rice while I was at Princeton. During my years as a graduate student at Rice, I worked as a research assistant for Thomas Cole, who introduced me to medical humanities as well as bioethics, and when I completed my dissertation he hired me (as assistant professor) in 2009 to teach in the McGovern Center for Humanities and Ethics at McGovern Medical School. Jeffrey Spike also was hired at the same time to work in the McGovern Center, and he mentored me in clinical ethics as my senior colleague.

A key theoretical—as well as personal—component of this book involves the thought of Paul Tillich, one of the most influential theologians of the last century. College was difficult for me in terms of my faith journey because of the material I was studying. I have written about this in *Religious Mourning: Reversals and Restorations of Psychological Portraits of Religious Leaders*,[1] and so I do not want to recount that narrative here. But suffice it to say that my undergraduate studies induced a crisis that was not resolved until I read Tillich's *Dynamics of Faith*.[2] Coincidently, Tillich also was very important to the development of pastoral theology. So Tillich holds a special place in my heart for many reasons.

I would like to thank Lucy Randall, editor at Oxford University Press, for believing in this project and for moving this book along through the production process from start to finish, as well as Hannah Doyle and Ayshwarya Ramakrishnan.

I also would like to thank my colleagues at the University of Texas Health Science Center at Houston (UTHealth), especially the core faculty and staff in the McGovern Center for Humanities and Ethics. They have been wonderful to work with over the years: Thomas Cole, Rebecca Lunstroth, Keisha Ray, Alma Rosas, and Angela Polczynski. Angela deserves a special word of thanks, because she proofread the text. Other colleagues in the McGovern Center who have influenced my thinking via discussions, seminars, and retreats include Samuel Karff, Jeffrey Spike, Eugene Boisaubin, Anson Koshy, Kirsten Ostherr, Cathy Rozmus, Deborah Franklin, Pedro Mancias, Eric Solberg, Sylvia Villarreal, Benjamin Saxton, Claire Clark, Woods Nash, Alina Bennett, Christine Wieseler, and Timothy Houk. I would like to thank William Howze for preparing the index and securing permissions.

I would like to thank Genevieve Cruz for sharing her de-identified clinical journals with me, as well as "Atlas" (not his real name), a medical resident who spent many hours with me in pastoral conversation.

Many parts of this book have been presented at various professional meetings.[3] Two groups in particular deserve special attention: the Group for New Directions in Pastoral Theology and the American Society for Bioethics and Humanities. Regarding the former, Robert Dykstra has been a constant source of support for me, reading my work more closely than any other person. Regarding the latter, Keith Meador has been a refreshing interlocutor in recent years.

Also, two colleagues provided extensive feedback on the substance of this book: Mindy McGarrah Sharp and Jon Wolfshohl. Mindy Sharp is a pastoral theologian (with training in clinical ethics), and Jon Wolfshohl is an emergency room physician (with a certificate in medical humanities). I invited both to read and to provide feedback on the complete manuscript prior to peer review. We spent two days together in Houston, Texas, discussing their feedback. I then revised the manuscript based on their comments. I paid for their time and travel via funds available in the Samuel Karff Chair. I would like to thank Thomas Cole for his leadership in creating this endowment and for nominating me to be a holder of the Chair. It is a deep honor to have this title.

Finally, I would like to dedicate this book to my wife, the Reverend Keatan King. Keatan is an endless source of love, laughter, fun, affirmation, affection, passion, kindness, creativity, stimulation, and encouragement. A devoted wife and an adoring mother, she has brought to me the most wonderful gift in the world, our darling daughter, Cohen May Carlin. Thank you, Keatan, for showing me that "adventure is out there"[4]! I am grateful that we are sharing the adventure together.

INTRODUCTION: BIOETHICS AND THEOLOGY

Definitions and conceptions of bioethics abound. Indeed, an online dictionary defines bioethics as "a field of study concerned with the ethics and philosophical implications of certain biological and medical procedures, technologies, and treatments, [such] as organ transplants, genetic engineering, and care of the terminally ill."[1] This definition is as good of a starting point as any for anyone seeking an introduction to the field. It offers a little more clarity than the suggestive etymological meaning of the word: bio (life) and ethics (the study of morality). A more robust definition of bioethics is offered in *The Encyclopedia of Bioethics*. The entry "bioethics" notes that bioethics "has come to encompass a number of fields and disciplines broadly grouped under the rubric *the life sciences*."[2] The entry goes on to distinguish a variety of bioethics: theoretical bioethics, clinical ethics, policy bioethics, and cultural bioethics. In a less authoritative book, though one much more creative than both the dictionary and the encyclopedia, titled *The Brewsters* (which is an introduction to bioethics for health professional students written in the genre of a choose-your-own-adventure novel), Jeffrey Spike asserts that bioethics consists of clinical ethics, professionalism, and research ethics.[3]

A common strategy for defining bioethics is by describing its origins. The concreteness of this approach helps readers to get a sense of the general questions of bioethics as well as its methods of inquiry and research. As a field, bioethics is often said to have originated in the United States during the mid- to late twentieth century after certain advances, scandals, paradoxes, and questions relating to clinical practice and biomedical research.[4] Albert Jonsen, who is not a trained historian but is one of the founders of bioethics as well as a Jesuit priest who taught for many years at the University of Washington in Seattle, Washington, recalls, "By the end of the

1970s, bioethics . . . [was] a new discipline with a distinctive literature and all the panoply of courses and conferences that academic disciplines engender."[5] Today bioethics is well established around the globe. There are departments and centers. There are groups and conferences and many subfields, including research ethics and public health ethics as well as different kinds of clinical ethics (e.g., psychiatric ethics, surgical ethics, nursing ethics, dental ethics, neuroethics, etc.).

Jonsen chronicles a number of issues and events from the 1940s through the 1980s that contributed to the conditions that enabled the emergence of bioethics. These include the Nuremberg trials during the mid-1940s in which Nazi physicians and administrators were tried on account of their roles in various murders and tortures during World War II; the discovery of the deoxyribonucleic acid (DNA) molecule, which was written about in an article by James Watson and Francis Crick in *Nature* on April 25, 1953,[6] raising new moral questions regarding genetics; the successful transplantation of a kidney by Dr. Joseph Murray and his team on December 23, 1954, which challenged some basic tenets of traditional medical ethics ("do no harm") in that a healthy twin was harmed because his kidney was removed and given to his twin brother; the approval of Enovid, an oral contraceptive ("the pill"), by the US Food and Drug Administration in 1960; the creation of the Admissions and Policy Committee of the Seattle Artificial Kidney Center after the successful launching of chronic dialysis treatment on March 9, 1960,[7] which set social worth criteria to determine who was eligible to receive this lifesaving procedure; the first heart transplantation by Dr. Christiaan Barnard on December 3, 1967[8]; the establishment of an ad hoc committee at Harvard Medical School that offered a new definition of death (brain death) in the *New England Journal of Medicine* on August 5, 1968,[9] which paved the way for more organ transplants; the publication of an article in the *New York Times* on July 26, 1972,[10] announcing that the US Public Health Service had been observing, but not treating, for forty years some four hundred African American patients who had been diagnosed with syphilis, even though an effective treatment for syphilis—penicillin—became widely available during the course of the study; a ruling by the US Supreme Court (*Roe v. Wade*) on January 22, 1973, which legalized abortion in certain circumstances; the ruling of the New Jersey Supreme Court on March 31, 1976, to allow life support to be withdrawn from Karen Ann Quinlan,[11] who, according to neurologists, was in a persistent vegetative state; the birth of Louise Brown on July 25, 1978,[12] by means of in vitro fertilization—the world's first "test tube baby"; the death of Baby Doe on April 15, 1980, when parents of a child born with Down syndrome elected to allow their child to die by refusing to permit surgeons to correct a blocked bowel—a relatively easy surgery to perform—because the parents did not want to raise a child with developmental disabilities, a decision to which President Ronald Reagan greatly objected; an operation performed by Dr. William DeVries on December 1, 1982, in which Barney Clark received an artificial heart, after which Clark lived for 112 days and became somewhat of a celebrity; and the publication of numerous articles that announced an AIDS epidemic in the early 1980s,[13] as well as a statement from the National Institutes of Health on the same day that it was suspected that a retrovirus caused the syndrome.[14] Nazis, DNA molecules, brain death, organ transplants, and test tube babies—this is the stuff of bioethics, at least as usually conceived, both by journalists and scholars. Bioethics, to many, is overwhelmingly sensational.

But it should be noted that telling the history of bioethics in this way is a political act. Storytelling[15] is a way of drawing attention to the field, articulating its importance, and generating profits. In *Observing Bioethics* Renée Fox and Judith Swazey illustrate the political nature of telling the history of fields by noting that, on September 23–24, 1992, Jonsen hosted a conference titled "The Birth of Bioethics" at the University of Washington on the occasion of the thirtieth anniversary of the publication of an article in *Life* that discussed the actions of the Admissions and Policy Committee of the Seattle Artificial Kidney Center.[16] Fox and Swazey point out: "Although he portrayed the events in Seattle as marking the start of bioethics in the United States, Jonsen acknowledged in a post-conference letter to the speakers that his identification of a specific birth date in part had the 'chauvinistic goal' of linking 'the events at [the] University of Washington with the beginnings of the field.'"[17]

Origin stories, Jonsen understood, serve particular ends, in this case the ends of placing the University of Washington (Jonsen's place of employment) at the center of bioethics. Fox and Swazey encourage us to be skeptical about not only Jonsen's origin story but also *all* origin stories, inviting us to ask: *Whose interests are being served by a given story?*

Fox and Swazey observe a number of origin stories of bioethics; the history of bioethics can be told in many ways. Some origin stories, they note, describe bioethics as the result of technological *advancements* (such as the invention of dialysis) while others focus on ethical *dilemmas* (such as confusion about birth control). Other origin stories emphasize historical *events* (such as the Nuremberg trials) while others highlight the founding of *organizations* (such as the Hastings Center). Still other origin stories underscore the coining of *terms* such as "bioethics." To be sure, many writers argue for "a multiyear, multicausal gestation" or, to put it more plainly, that many issues and events contributed to the emergence of bioethics, the view that Fox and Swazey favor.[18] It seems hard to disagree with such a reasonable perspective.

The Secularization of Bioethics

The way I like the story of bioethics told, because I am a religious person, emphasizes the role of theological thinkers in the founding of the field. Lisa Cahill, a theologian, tells a version of this story well.[19] She notes that the vast majority of those who first published in bioethics had theological training, including Paul Ramsey, Richard McCormick, and James Gustafson—perhaps the three most notable scholars of the early years—as well as Joseph Fletcher, Karen Lebacqz, Fred Rosner, Immanuel Jakobvitz, Elliot Dorff, and David Bleich. In a footnote she adds that a number of students of Gustafson entered the field early on, including James Childress, Allen Verhey, Stanley Hauerwas, and Margaret Farley. She lists others as well, such as David Smith, Warren Reich, Charles Curran, William May, and Robert Veatch. All of this is to say that, as Cahill chronicles here, theologians or scholars with theological and/or religious studies training played a very important role in the founding and in the developing of bioethics; philosophers, lawyers, and others entered bioethics a little later. But as bioethics established itself some felt that public debates about bioethics needed to be nonsectarian and to occur on so-called neutral ground. So the early theologically trained bioethicists translated their insights regarding moral matters into a secular language, most often with the application of abstract principles.[20] Jonsen writes personally in a book chapter about how he did exactly this when he took a position at a medical school.[21]

Daniel Callahan, cofounder of the Hastings Center, tells a similar story to Cahill's in a 1990 commentary titled "Religion and the Secularization of Bioethics":

> The most striking change over the past two decades or so has been the secularization of bioethics. The field has moved from one dominated by religious and medical traditions to one now increasingly shaped by philosophical and legal concepts. The consequence has been a mode of public discourse that emphasizes secular themes: universal rights, individual self-direction, procedural justice, and a systematic denial of either a common good or a transcendent individual good.[22]

He also notes that when he first became interested in bioethics in the mid-1960s that the only resources available were "theological or those drawn from within the traditions of medicine, themselves heavily shaped by religion."[23] But, in time, theologians left the field. Callahan offers two contributing factors: (i) theologians and religious studies scholars became more interested in discussions of race and class in the 1970s (to contemporary readers familiar with the history of religious studies it is noticeable that he does not mention gender) and (ii) as bioethics became established in the public sphere, "there was great pressure (even if more latent than manifest) to frame the issues, and to speak, in a common secular mode."[24] He adds:

> I do not want to imply that there was any outright hostility toward religion (even though I could detect that now and then in some philosophers I knew). On the contrary, it [religion] was for the most part bypassed altogether. . . . There was (and still is) a lurking fear of religion, often seen as a source of deep and unresolvable moral conflict.[25]

An illustration of the trend to find a common secular mode of discourse can be observed in the Belmont Report, which was published by the US Department of Health, Education, and Welfare on April 18, 1979.[26] This report was commissioned after the scandal of the Tuskegee Syphilis Study.[27] A general feeling in the United States emerged then that scientists and researchers no longer could be trusted to be left alone to do their work, that guidelines and protections were needed, and that racism and various abuses of power were too vast and too deep to ignore. Since the 1970s, many shocking exposés have been written about the history of clinical experiments on vulnerable populations, such as Allen Hornblum's *Acres of Skin: Human Experiments at Holmesburg Prison*, a book that recounts the systematic practices of exploitation by physicians and scientists who viewed the prisoners as an endless supply of skin for their dermatological research.[28]

The bulk of the Belmont Report was written by Tom Beauchamp. Beauchamp, who received a Bachelor of Divinity degree from Yale Divinity School in 1966 (yet another example of a founder of bioethics having had theological training) and a Doctor of Philosophy degree from Johns Hopkins University in 1970, was working at the time as a staff member for the National Institutes of Health. According to Beauchamp, on a retreat together the commission agreed on three principles that were to guide human subjects research. These principles were felt to be nonsectarian and thus suitable for public policy. The principles were: respect for persons, beneficence, and justice. The assignment given to Beauchamp was to spell out what these principles mean and to explain how they relate to each other, so as to guide future research.

Beauchamp asked his supervisor what these principles in the Belmont Report mean. His supervisor replied that he did not know and the commission also probably did not know either, so he advised Beauchamp to take a prospective (not a retrospective) view on the principles. In other words, he encouraged Beauchamp to take this as an opportunity to shape the future direction of the field.[29]

He did. Indeed, Beauchamp (with James Childress) went on to publish *Principles of Biomedical Ethics*,[30] a work that became the most widely cited book in bioethics, in which a method that came to be known as principlism was advocated. In the book Beauchamp and Childress rephrased a principle from the Belmont Report (respect for persons became respect for autonomy), and they added a fourth principle (nonmaleficence). Also, they theorized and applied these four principles—respect for autonomy, nonmaleficence, beneficence, and justice—in a much more extended fashion than was possible in the brief government report. Strikingly, these principles later spread to other health professions as bioethics continued to gain ground (e.g., Phyllis Beemsterboer applied these principles to dental hygiene[31]).

The work of Beauchamp and Childress has been criticized by many.[32] Some critiques will be explored in subsequent chapters. But whatever one may think of *Principles of Biomedical Ethics*, one must nevertheless engage it in the field of bioethics because it is so influential. Indeed, this book is the starting point for anyone entering the field. And, for anyone re-envisioning the field, as I am attempting to do in this book in a modest way, one would be hard-pressed to pick a better starting point than *Principles of Biomedical Ethics*.

Recovering Religion in Bioethics

Over the last decade or so there has been a recovery of theological thinking in bioethics and related areas, as evidenced by, for example, the John Templeton Foundation and others providing generous funding to the University of Chicago to launch the Program on Religion and Medicine in 2009. This program provides a number of venues for studying religion and medicine, including an annual conference. Also, the Institute for Spirituality and Health (ISH) in Houston, Texas, which is a part of the Texas Medical Center (TMC), has been an important institution dedicated to attending to matters of religion, faith, spirituality, and the health professions, providing various platforms for scholarly activity. The ISH, like the Hastings Center, was an important early institution in helping to establish bioethics as a field. Of note, the ISH hosts an annual conference on the theme of psychotherapy and faith.[33]

Another way that theological thinking has been recovered in bioethics is by means of publications. A significant volume in this regard is David Guinn's *Handbook of Bioethics and Religion*.[34] This edited collection directly challenges the notion that bioethics should—or can—be neutral. On this point Guinn quotes Michael McConnell: "In the marketplace of ideas, secular viewpoints and ideologies are in competition with religious viewpoints and ideologies. It is no more neutral to favor the secular over the religious than it is to favor the religious over the secular."[35] Relatedly, because postmodern, feminist, womanist, and other contextual thinkers in various disciplines have challenged the concept of "objectivity," the door has been opened for theological or religious perspectives in various intellectual and political arenas, including bioethics.[36] Cahill has written,

> Theologians searching for a new model of thinking bioethically should recall postmodernism's insight that even abstract and supposedly universal principles always come to be articulated out of particular and historical communities of practice and discernment. Every political value system or agenda has a past, a context, and a set of investments, whether it be liberal democracy, the scientific research imperative, free market economics, communitarianism, or socialism.[37]

She adds: "Context-generated moral insights and proposals can gain a public hearing if they can prove themselves relevant and useful in the various contexts that together make up the common good of interest to the public in question."[38] In other words, to exclude religious perspectives from bioethics would be arbitrary just as it would be arbitrary to exclude perspectives derived from, say, preference utilitarianism. Thus, the door has been opened—or, rather, reopened—for theological or religious perspectives in bioethics, which is one reason why the number of books, articles, and journals offering particular religious perspectives on bioethics is growing.[39]

What This Book Adds

This book is different from what is usually thought of as theological bioethics. What this books adds—how it is different from most accounts of theological bioethics—is that this is a work of what I call *pastoral aesthetics*. I will unpack what I mean by this term in chapter 1. But suffice it to say that the distinguishing feature of this book is its employment of pastoral theology (via a distinct interdisciplinary method of correlation) in bioethics.

A related book to this one is Sondra Ely Wheeler's *Stewards of Life: Bioethics and Pastoral Care*.[40] She, too, engages Beauchamp and Childress's four principles of bioethics from a theological perspective—what I do in this book—but an important difference is that she does so as a theological ethicist, not as a pastoral theologian. Thus, the subtitle of her book is somewhat of a misnomer. She examines Beauchamp and Childress's principles in context of and also in tension with Christian understandings of the moral life, the upshot being that "the substantive meanings of qualities like justice or beneficence must be constructed: they are hardly evident in terms themselves" and that "the notion of universal, belief-neutral principles which have only to be applied to new situations to yield moral clarity is itself illusory."[41] As a theological ethicist, Wheeler uses specific passages from the Bible, especially the New Testament, as well as particular Christian doctrines, such as teachings on suffering, to engage Beauchamp and Childress's principles. This is a common way of doing Christian bioethics.[42]

A Sample Argument in Theological Ethics

Let me offer a brief example of how arguments in theological ethics are often made. In *Bioethics: A Primer for Christians*, Gilbert Meilaender points out that although "a great deal of the best work in bioethics has involved the application of certain ethical principles—such as respect for autonomy, beneficence, and justice—to particular issues of concern, there is no way to apply principles in a vacuum."[43] He continues: "How we understand such principles, and how we understand the situations we encounter, will depend on background beliefs that we bring to moral reflection—beliefs about the meaning of human life, the significance of suffering and dying, and the ultimate context in which to understand our being and doing."[44] These background beliefs, Meilaender suggests, often are not the product of reasoned argument, for they are what he calls "prearticulate."[45]

Terms such as background beliefs and prearticulate recall a common way of distinguishing morality and ethics where morality is what a person is taught about right and wrong (and is, therefore, a product of one's upbringing and culture) and ethics, as an academic discipline, is, to use Meilaender's term, "reasoned argument" concerning morality. In other words, morality is assumed whereas ethics is argued. Or, to put it another way, ethics is the study of morality.[46]

In his primer Meilaender offers some basic moral assumptions held by many Christians that he believes should guide Christians as they think about issues in bioethics, with the purpose of demonstrating a contrast to secular approaches in bioethics, especially principlist approaches. Principlist bioethics has been criticized for privileging the principle of respect for autonomy. Meilaender joins this criticism: "We should not suppose that any individual's dignity can be satisfactorily described by the language of autonomy alone—as if we were most fully human when we acted on our own, chose the course of our 'life plan,' or were capable and powerful enough to burden no one."[47] Meilaender wants to be clear that, if the dominant paradigm in bioethics—or at least certain (mis)interpretations of the dominant paradigm in bioethics—assumes the primacy of autonomy, he does not believe that Christian bioethics should affirm this assumption.

Other key components of Meilaender's particular Christian moral vision include the following notions: human beings are both free and finite; human beings are both persons and bodies; suffering, while not good in itself, is not to be avoided at all costs; and health, while a good (health is something to be pursued), is not the supreme good (i.e., health is not something to be pursued at *all* costs). These moral assumptions inform his assessment of many issues in bioethics, including human reproduction, abortion, genetics, euthanasia, organ donation, and human subjects research. Such is the scope of Meilaender's primer. And what this primer does, as all theological accounts of bioethics do, is offer a particular vision of moral living with regard to the health sciences.

How Meilaender's theological bioethics works can be illustrated by focusing on a particular issue, such as, say, abortion. Meilaender notes that, while the issue of abortion has been very divisive for decades, "for Christians, this issue should be relatively straightforward."[48] He adds: "We know what we ought to do, but we find it hard to act in accord with that knowledge. If many Christians have nonetheless become unsure about the morality of abortion, that lack of clarity represents our failure in the face of pressure from the surrounding culture."[49] His position on abortion, as one might surmise from reading these quotations, is that abortion is wrong. I should note that I am not advocating Meilaender's vision; in what follows I am describing it for illustrative purposes.

How does Meilaender ground his argument? He begins by suggesting that Christians historically have been against abortion, in contrast to dominant voices within the Roman Empire. For evidence he cites an early Christian text—the *Didache*—that condemns abortion. He also cites scripture (e.g., Psalm 139:13–16), as well as church doctrine on Christology where it is taught that "in Jesus of Nazareth God has lived and redeemed the entirety of human life, from its very beginnings to the death toward which we all go," and that Christ "has been with us in the darkness of the womb as he will be in the darkness of the tomb."[50] Arguments in theological ethics, then, usually consist of citations, syntheses, and applications of various sources of Christian tradition, such as historical practice, biblical witness, and church teaching.

Human experience as well as insights and findings from nontheological fields and disciplines can inform theological ethics as well. Arguments in theological ethics also often engage moral philosophy. With regard to abortion, an important category emphasized by feminist ethicists in recent decades is "personhood," where it is argued that embryos and fetuses do not have moral value (or at least not the same moral value) as children and adults because embryos and fetuses lack or appear to lack certain capacities, such as consciousness. Meilaender rejects such arguments:

> Popular as such "personhood" arguments have become, they have obvious difficulties which occur to almost everyone who considers them. In particular, these arguments often raise "slippery slope" worries for us. If they justify abortion, may they not justify considerably more as well? . . . [T]here will be newborns, many senile [*sic*] elderly people, and some retarded [*sic*] people who do not qualify as "persons" and who therefore do not have as strong a claim upon us for protection and care as full-fledged persons do. And, indeed, one philosopher [Mary Anne Warren], pressing such an argument in an oft-cited article, once suggested that a fetus could have no more right to life than a newborn guppy.[51]

In short, Meilaender offers a Christian bioethics of abortion that employs sources of moral authority—such as tradition and scripture—and also attacks philosophical arguments that attempt to justify abortion. This, in terms of structure, is a good illustration of how arguments in theological ethics are made.

But it is important to emphasize that within Christianity different persons hold radically different moral assumptions. For instance, feminist theological ethicists Beverly Harrison and Shirley Cloyes write that, while in Christian theology life is a gift from God, "the elevation of procreation as the central symbol of divine benevolence happened over time. . . . It did not, for instance, typify the very early, primitive Christian community. The synoptic gospels provide ample evidence that procreation played no such metaphorical role in early Christianity."[52]

This elevation, they argue, occurred later, and for patriarchal reasons. As the early Christian movement became a religion, men assumed more authority, crafting doctrine that functioned in a sexist way. Harrison and Cloyes, then, offer a critical assessment of church tradition, one in direct conflict with Meilaender's, leading them to conclude:

> We desperately need a desacralization of our biological power to reproduce and at the same time a real concern for human dignity and the social conditions for personhood and the values of human relationship. And note that the desacralization does not mean complete devaluation of the worth of procreation. It means we must shift away from the notion that the central metaphors for divine blessing are expressed at the biological level to the recognition that our social relations bear the image of what is most holy.[53]

Harrison and Cloyes continue, "Professional male Christian ethicists [like Meilaender] tend to assume that Christianity has an unbroken history of 'all but absolute' prohibition of abortion and that the history of morality of abortion can best be traced by studying the teaching of the now best-remembered theologians."[54]

The upshot of this brief discussion of Meilaender's primer is this: the same critique he offers of principlist bioethics—there is no way to apply moral principles in a vacuum—applies to his own vision of Christian bioethics. *There is no way to apply material from Christian sources (*e.g., *scripture) in a vacuum.* Harrison and Cloyes's assessment of abortion illustrates this (they are Christian *and* they are prochoice, as are many liberal Christians). Moreover, a large body of literature has emerged in recent decades, making this point with regard to biblical interpretation: there is no view from nowhere or some universal way to interpret texts, experiences, and issues.[55]

In contrast to Meilaender and Wheeler, this book does not take traditional religious sources of moral authority such as the Bible and use these sources to answer questions raised by bioethics, the most common way of relating religion and bioethics. Rather, in this book I engage images of pastoral care. This is because a common starting point for pastoral theology, unlike theological ethics, is human experience. Some readers may find themselves surprised by how little religion, as usually understood, is in the book. Also, because mainstream bioethics is often sensational, this book focuses more (though not exclusively) on the mundane. It focuses less on brain death and kidney transplants and more on the little ways individuals find themselves crushed by the forces of modern medicine.

Another Book on Principlist Bioethics?

I realize that some readers may feel that what bioethics as a field needs is something entirely brand new, not another book engaging *Principles of Biomedical Ethics*. Moreover, because *Principles of Biomedical Ethics* has many critics (and the criticisms of principlism are well known), even a book deconstructing *Principles of Biomedical Ethics* would seem to be redundant as well. However, what I offer in this book is an embracing of *and* a rejection of *Principles of Biomedical Ethics*. A goal of this book is to convince critics of principlism that the principles have more to offer than is commonly realized and that pastoral theology has something to contribute to principlist bioethics that is satisfying for its critics and fans alike.

The Organization of This Book

This book is organized according to the four principles in *Principles of Biomedical Ethics*. Chapter 1 focuses on correlational methodology, and then chapters 2, 3, 4, and 5 each focus on one of the principles of Beauchamp and Childress, as correlated with one of four images of pastoral care. Chapter 2 correlates the principle of respect for autonomy with the image of the living human document. Chapter 3 correlates the principle of nonmaleficence with the image of the circus clown. Chapter 4 correlates the principle of beneficence with the image of the diagnostician. Chapter 5 correlates the principle of justice with the image the living human web. The epilogue of the book addresses contemporary issues of pluralism and spiritualty and also offers some final thoughts on future possibilities raised by the implications of this book.

1 PRINCIPLIST BIOETHICS AND PASTORAL THEOLOGY

The central claim of this book is that pastoral theologians can bring something distinctive to bioethics. Specifically, pastoral theologians can enrich moral imagination in bioethics by cultivating an aesthetic sensibility that is theologically-informed, psychologically-sophisticated, therapeutically-oriented, and experientially-grounded. This book provides "a way of looking at things,"[1] which, influenced by Robert Dykstra,[2] I call "pastoral aesthetics." In broader ethics literature, this book may be understood as contributing to what Kwame Appiah describes as our "moral intuitions," which "are often more secure than the principles we appeal to in explaining them."[3] This book does not offer new principles but rather a new way of looking at the ones that have formed and remain prominent in the field of bioethics.

Such inquiry in pastoral aesthetics can be accomplished in various ways. One way is that pastoral theologians can offer their own analysis of issues raised by bioethicists.[4] Another way is that scholars writing in bioethics can draw on the work of pastoral theologians who write about illness.[5] And yet another way is that pastoral theologians can expand and enrich the range of moral consideration in bioethics by suggesting new issues for bioethicists to consider.

This chapter will do several things. It begins with a discussion of principlism, focusing on its limits, thereby providing an opening for pastoral theology to contribute to bioethics. It then discusses several definitions of pastoral theology, giving special attention to various ways theology and psychology may be related in pastoral theology. A specific vision of pastoral theology is offered (pastoral theology as aesthetic imagination) as well as a means of positioning bioethics and pastoral theology (a method of correlation informed by art theory). The chapter closes with a discussion of images and ethics.

Principlism

Principles of Biomedical Ethics, as noted, is the most-cited book in bioethics.[6] No other book in bioethics has had comparable influence. Now in its seventh edition, Tom Beauchamp and James Childress write in the preface that when the book first went to press in 1977 both the field and the term "bioethics" were new. There was no way for the authors to know then that they were writing such an important book. While each edition has seen major changes, the book has kept intact its main structure, thus preserving what has become known as "the four-principles approach" or "principlism."[7] It is important to note, however, that, as Childress points out, "no single approach can be called *the* principles approach," because there are multiple principles-based approaches.[8] In this book I will refer to the work of Beauchamp and Childress in a variety of ways, but I prefer the term "principlist bioethics" because the other terms do not make it clear to persons outside of the field that these terms are approaches to decision-making specifically within bioethics. Also, the term "principlist" has been invoked as a criticism of their work, so my use of the term implies a recognition on my part of the limits of their approach.

What is principlist bioethics? Principlist bioethics, as articulated by Beauchamp and Childress, offers a framework[9] of moral norms based on four principles that derive from common morality. Common morality is defined as core tenets about right and wrong that some believe are universal; it is asserted that these tenets emerged over the course of history and have been transmitted by means of communities.[10] Beauchamp and Childress do not claim to have identified all of these tenets. Rather, they offer four principles as a framework for identifying and analyzing ethical dilemmas in clinical practice as well as in scientific research. The four principles are respect for autonomy, beneficence, nonmaleficence, and justice. "That these four clusters of moral principles are central to biomedical ethics is a conclusion the authors of this work have reached," Beauchamp and Childress write, "by examining *considered moral judgements* and *the way moral beliefs cohere*."[11]

Principles are more concrete than theories (such as deontology and utilitarianism) but less specific than rules (such as do not lie and do not steal). Principlist bioethics offers a means of engaging ethical issues and dilemmas, which are assessed by specifying[12] the content of the principles in a given context, and if the principles seem to conflict with each other, the dilemma is resolved by weighing and balancing the principles, determining which is more important.

In the preface to the seventh edition, Beauchamp and Childress address what has been a persistent—and, in their view, misguided—criticism of their work:

> Many have suggested . . . that, in line with what they perceive as an American individualist orientation, the principle of respect for autonomy dominates and overrides all other moral principles and considerations in our work. This interpretation of our book is profoundly mistaken. . . . We have always argued that many kinds of competing moral considerations validly override this principle under certain conditions. Examples include the following: if our choices endanger public health potentially harm innocent others, or require a scarce and unfunded resource, others can justifiably restrict our exercises of autonomy.[13]

They add that "it is a mistake in biomedical ethics to assign priority to any basic principle over other basic principles," and that "the better strategy is to appreciate both the contributions and the limits of various principles, virtues, and rights, which is the strategy we adopt."[14] It is important to note, too, that others have suggested different or additional principles than those offered by Beauchamp and Childress, such as veracity.[15]

Beauchamp and Childress are right that their work has been unfairly criticized with regard to the principle of respect for autonomy. However, there have been a number of other critiques raised about their approach that do have considerable merit (some of these will be explored in subsequent chapters). One that is especially important for my argument in this book may be put as follows: *principlist bioethics pays insufficient attention to experience and to context.* While principlist bioethics does in fact tend to be detached and abstract, pastoral theology can supplement principlist bioethics by paying more attention to experience and to context. What is offered in this book, therefore, is not only a critique of principlist bioethics but also a critique of the criticism of principlist bioethics, for principlist bioethics can be richer than is often assumed.

Experiential and Contextual Critiques of Principlist Bioethics

Further discussion of this experiential and contextual critique of principlist bioethics is in order, both so that it can be properly understood and so that the contributions of pastoral theology can become clearer. One scholar who has offered this critique of mainstream bioethics is Richard Miller. Miller notes that bioethics tends to be more philosophical than ethnographic and that sociologists and anthropologists lament that "conventional bioethics fails to explore the social contours and experiential complexities of professional life."[16] Miller continues: "Excluded from the standard account of bioethics are medical professionals' moral idioms, personal challenges, logistical obstacles, religious commitments, and interpersonal interactions with patients and families."[17] He adds: "Instead, medical ethics is often abstract, deductive, and/or highly rationalistic, detached from the anguishing empirical realities and power struggles in which medical professionals find themselves."[18] In support of this critique, Miller cites the work of Arthur Kleinman, who similarly argues that conventional bioethics "fails to capture the existential challenges of patient suffering."[19] Kleinman is disappointed that "lay perspectives" and "everyday life experiences" are not central in bioethics.[20]

William Branch offers a similar critique. "The traditional triad of principles—beneficence, autonomy, and justice—is very familiar to anyone who has sat in a class on medical ethics," he writes, and "we teach our future doctors to solve ethical dilemmas by juggling the weights of these three principles."[21] Branch derides this approach as "detached." An example of such detached medical ethics can be observed in one of the earliest textbooks of the field, by Albert Jonsen, Mark Siegler, and William Winslade, titled *Clinical Ethics*:

> A 74-year-old man with chronic pulmonary disease is admitted in mild respiratory failure and with diffuse bronchospasm. His respiratory condition probably does not require emergency intubation. The therapeutic options include medical management and observation in an effort to avoid or postpone intubation. After considering the situation, the chief resident orders early intubation, and one of the reasons for this choice is to allow an inexperienced intern to practice intubating a patient.[22]

This tendency toward abstraction persists in contemporary textbooks. Indeed, in perhaps the most widely used clinical ethics textbook today, Bernard Lo's *Resolving Ethical Dilemmas*, there is this case:

> A 32-year old man with a positive test for human immunodeficiency virus (HIV) antibodies refuses to notify his wife. "If she finds out, it would destroy our marriage." Should the physician notify the wife despite the patient's objections? Although maintaining patient confidentiality is important, it seems cruel not to warn the wife that she is at risk for a fatal infection. What are the reasons that justify the physician's decision?[23]

These examples, from an early textbook and a contemporary one, are not examples of principlist bioethics per se but rather a common tendency in bioethics, though, it should be noted, Beauchamp and Childress offered an appendix of such cases in the first edition of their book.[24] In response to this tendency, whole subfields have emerged (such as narrative medicine[25]) that attempt to add more flavor, depth, and complexity to bioethics by paying closer attention to context and experience.

When scholars such as Miller and Kleinman use terms and phrases such as "conventional bioethics" and "the standard account of bioethics," it is quite often principlist bioethics to which they are referring. John Barbour offers a similar critique as Miller's and in doing so explicitly criticizes principlist bioethics:

> The principles-based paradigm of ethical reflection that has dominated the field since the 1960s is said to the isolate the quandary, the moment of difficult ethical choice, from the larger temporal context of a patient's life. A second criticism is that the concern to protect patient autonomy severs our understanding of persons from the communities and relationships that give their lives meaning.[26]

"Current paradigms of bioethics," Barbour continues, "also obscure both the bodily basis of self-identity and the soul—patients' deepest sense of their lives' meaning. And the religious values that should guide ethical reflection are slighted when the overriding goal is to formulate a public policy or procedure that everyone in a pluralistic society can agree on."[27] He adds: "Moral reflection on medicine must not only consider dilemmas involved in restoring patients to physical health but also ill persons' and their caregivers' understanding of the meaning of life and death."[28] To do bioethics well, Barbour argues, one needs to take more seriously the *bio* in bioethics, and he suggests that a promising way to do this is by using more autobiography in bioethics, in conjunction with other ways of thinking about ethics. "Among the genres of narrative," he writes, "autobiography has a special kind of power and persuasiveness because of its claim to truthfulness, its capacity for detail, its expansive temporal context, its interest in revealing both individual character and the cultural forces that shape character, and its freedom to encompass both plotted events and topical or thematic discussion of ideas."[29]

This perspective, which favors autobiography, has generated a large body of literature that is referred to as "pathography."[30] The strength of this approach, in contrast to the brief three or four sentence cases offered previously, is that pathographies provide book-length discussions of single cases, long narratives of an encounter with an illness, raising many issues for moral consideration. Principlist bioethics, to be sure, could offer book-length discussions of single cases, but it has not done so. This book, while also not offering a book-length discussion of a single case, will draw on a number of pathographies.

Feminist critiques of principlist bioethics also focus on experience and context, with special attention being given to the perspectives and experiences of women. In *An Invitation to Feminist Ethics*, Hilde Lindemann notes that Carol Gilligan's[31] critique of Lawrence Kohlberg's[32] stage theory of moral development is grounded in the fact that (i) Kohlberg created a model based on the study of men and (ii) women, who do a great deal more of caregiving than men do in the United States even whether or not this work is paid,[33] tend to have a different moral orientation than men do due to their roles as caregivers. This difference, however, is not essential, and it is not universal. Yet this difference has practical implications. In response to feminist critque Beauchamp and Childress have integrated some insights from feminist ethicists in various editions of *Principles of Biomedical Ethics.*[34]

Having discussed important critiques of principlist bioethics, I now want to turn to recent calls in bioethics for more psychology that can help to address these critiques because various schools of psychology specialize in understanding human experience, and to do psychology well, social context cannot be ignored.

Recent Calls for More Psychology in Bioethics

In "Toward a Psychodynamic Approach to Bioethics," Jacob Appel notes that many of the first-generation bioethicists were psychiatrists and that some, such as William Gaylin (the cofounder of the Hastings Center), received psychoanalytic training. Yet bioethics developed largely apart from psychodynamic theory. So in this article, Appel calls for "a psychodynamic theory of bioethics."[35]

What might psychoanalysis add to bioethics? Appel observes that "personal attitudes regarding the most basic bioethical quandaries, such as the starting and ending points of life, cannot be explained solely through the sheer force of deductive logic."[36] On this point, many bioethicists agree. Indeed, in recent decades inductive approaches have flourished in bioethics.[37] Appel argues psychoanalysis can provide new understandings of moral disagreement both at theoretical levels (e.g., fierce debates among scholars regarding the ethics of abortion) and at clinical levels (e.g., heated arguments among family members during end-of-life decision-making). How? Citing Theodor Adorno, Appel suggestively notes that "the superego [can sometimes become] the spokesman of the id."[38] He explains:

> If the fundamental premises underlying personal attitudes toward bioethical issues are impenetrable to rational interrogation, but the conclusions derived from these premises are dressed-up in academic terminology and draped with secondary analysis, then an analogous phenomenon is occurring: a decision is being made or a conclusion being drawn for unconscious reasons, motivated by the id, and then the superego is cloaking these beliefs in a manner palatable to the psyche.[39]

Appel continues: "Bioethics largely ignores the century of literature relating to the underlying psychosexual desires of childhood"[40] and adds that many situations in clinical settings could be richly engaged with psychoanalytic insights: Oedipal issues relating to withdrawing treatment for a parent on life support; sibling rivalry issues in which one sibling is called upon to donate a kidney for another; and transference issues relating to the advice offered by a clinical ethicist. Appel also notes that the hospital setting is a dream-like space[41] and that conversations with clinical ethicists resemble conversations with therapists. While noting many issues that could be explored with psychoanalytic hermeneutics, Appel "makes no claim to develop a psychodynamic theory of bioethics" but emphasizes that "such a framework for analyzing bioethical dilemmas should be developed."[42]

Others, too, have called for more psychological contributions to bioethics, notably Thomas Murray, who has served as president of the American Society for Bioethics and Humanities as well as the Hastings Center. Murray has called for "bringing psychology into intimate and sustained dialogue with bioethics."[43] Murray, whose doctoral training was in social psychology, notes that only a few psychologists have made the journey to prominence in bioethics. He adds that there are exceptions (such as Ruth Faden and Adrienne Asch), but from his early days at the Hastings Center as a postdoctoral fellow, he does not recall many psychologists being present at the Hastings Center. Now, reflecting on his career and on the field, he feels that psychology can add a great deal, but, unlike Appel, Murray is not making a case for a specific school of psychology.

Yet it is important to point out that psychology is not completely absent in medical education or in bioethics—far from it. Indeed, all medical schools have courses (or course content) on behavioral medicine in which many issues in psychology are addressed, such as life cycle theory and various psychopathological disorders.[44] In clinical clerkships, "how to break bad news" sessions are common,[45] in which psychological dynamics are discussed. Moreover, the biopsychosocial approach to medicine has been widely advocated for decades, which, as its title intimates, includes psychology.[46] While it would be misleading to suggest that psychology is a complete stranger to medical education, ethics education in medical schools, and bioethics, Appel and Murray, who are quite familiar with medical education and bioethics literature, nevertheless are calling for a more systematic and thoroughgoing use of psychology.

The Opening for Pastoral Theology in Bioethics

To recap, if a major critique of principlist bioethics is its tendency to pay insufficient attention to experience and context, to remedy this deficiency scholars writing from literary and anthropological perspectives have employed methodologies beyond philosophy to do bioethics in a way that pays more attention to "thickness."[47] But literary and anthropological perspectives do not tend to draw on psychological theories and therapeutic techniques, which is why some bioethicists have called for more psychology in bioethics. Additionally, in recent years there has been a rebirth of religious perspectives in bioethics. Thus, what is being called for now from different places in bioethics is more psychology and more religion. Because the academic field most closely identified with psychology and religion is pastoral theology,[48] pastoral theologians have a special opportunity to contribute bioethics. This book emerges out of these criticisms and calls.

What Is Pastoral Theology?

Pastoral theology most simply defined is the theological discipline that provides the theory that informs practices, broadly conceived, of pastoral care, also broadly conceived.[49] James Dittes, who taught pastoral theology at Yale University for his whole academic career, once defined pastoral psychology as psychology from the pastor's point of view.[50] Following the same logic, pastoral theology can be thought of as theology from the pastor's point of view.

Historically, pastoral theology has had a special relationship with psychology in that psychological theories, such as those of Sigmund Freud and Carl Rogers, have informed the theories and methods of pastoral care and counseling.[51] Also, pastoral theology can be distinguished from other forms of theology such as systematic theology. While systematic theology examines how different doctrines (such as, say, predestination and atonement) fit together logically, pastoral theology is concerned less with coherence than function. That is to say, whereas systematic theology often is concerned with how doctrines relate to one another, pastoral theology focuses on how doctrines operate in the lives of individuals, in the life of the church, and in communities beyond the church walls.

Pastoral theology sometimes can be in tension with systematic theology. In *Images of Pastoral Care: Classic Readings*, Dykstra offers a conversation overheard by pastoral theologian Valerie DeMarinis between two professors of systematic theology who were denigrating pastoral theology:

> They are just like scavengers. They have no real theory, just a hunting and pecking, a grabbing and applying. There is no order for them. And they can never explain what they do or why they do it, only that something works or not. It is all technique, and at best has some rationale to measure if it works. It is a very sad state of affairs.[52]

Dykstra notes that DeMarinis, first troubled by this conversation, came to embrace the image of the scavenger because scavengers are highly skilled: "The responsible scavenger," she writes, "is one skilled at survival, one who knows how to search, salvage, purify, and transform the elements of the world into that which nurtures and sustains life."[53] DeMarinis reframed this insult as a compliment.

The *Dictionary of Pastoral Care and Counseling* has several entries related to defining pastoral theology.[54] One of them (on Protestant pastoral theology) is coauthored by J. R. Burck and Rodney Hunter.[55] They note that while there is no consensus on the definition of pastoral theology there are three definitions that are readily identifiable: (i) "the branch of theology that formulates the practical principles, theories, and procedures for ordained ministry in all of its functions (though in the nineteenth century often excluding homiletics)"; (ii) "the practical theological discipline concerned with the theory and practice of pastoral care and counseling"; and (iii) "a form of theological reflection in which pastoral experience serves as a context for the critical development of basic theological understanding." Regarding the third definition, Burck and Hunter add,

> Pastoral theology in this sense generally focuses on topics like illness, death, sexuality, family, and personhood, though in principle any theology topic may be considered *from a pastoral perspective*—faith, hope, love, salvation, and God, for example. Here pastoral theology is not a theology *of* or *about* pastoral care but a type of contextual theology [like black theology, feminist theology, womanist theology, liberation theology, etc.], a way of doing theology *pastorally*.[56]

In the entry there is also a subsection on theology and ethics, in which it is noted that pastoral theology "is distinguished from systematic theology and ethics with regard to both concreteness and practicality, for systematics and ethics are primarily concerned with articulating and critically developing general meanings and principles" and that, while pastoral theology also always deals with normative claims and issues, there is little consensus about "how normative visions relate to practical and empirical analyses."[57] Burck and Hunter point out that some, such as Don Browning,[58] see pastoral theology as a branch of ethics (thus centralizing the role of normative perspectives in pastoral theology) while others, such as James Lapsley,[59] "feel that this approach [i.e., Browning's] overstresses normative reflection at the expense of the analysis of actual human dynamics, the discipline's most distinctive and valuable point of contribution."[60] This basic disagreement has generated a large body of literature on the relationship between theology and psychology.[61]

In this book, I side with Lapsley and others who feel that Browning overstresses normative reflection at the expense of the analysis of human experience. Why? For my purposes in this book, it would be odd to endorse a normative version of pastoral theology (i.e., Browning's) in bioethics because such a path would have less to offer bioethics; what bioethics needs, again, is not more attention to normative reflection but more attention to human experience. Finally, I would like to add that the vision of pastoral theology that I previously outlined is my own take on the field; there are other ways to conceive of the field.[62]

Pastoral Theology as Aesthetic Imagination

In this book I affirm the third definition of pastoral theology previously offered: "a form of theological reflection in which pastoral experience serves as a context for the critical development of basic theological understanding." Specifically, I view pastoral theology as a form of what Dykstra has called "aesthetic imagination."[63] What Dykstra means by this will be unpacked in the following discussion.

In the introduction of *Images of Pastoral Care*, Dykstra sketches out a vision of and for pastoral theology. He begins by recounting the origins of the field and notes that the founder of pastoral theology, Anton Boisen, created Clinical Pastoral Education (CPE) to be a training program for seminary students to gain experience in specialized settings such as hospitals. He adds that Boisen spent a considerable amount of time in inpatient psychiatric care not only as a caregiver but also as a patient (Boisen was diagnosed with schizophrenia). Dykstra suggests that pastoral theology in its very founding is *unstable*, like Boisen's mental constitution: "Pastoral theology was born of madness and, one could argue, has yet to fully recover. A fragile, sometimes fragmented identity on the margins of church and society seems to be its peculiar portion and destiny."[64]

Dykstra adds: "In practical terms this means that pastoral theologians . . . have rarely felt terribly certain of just who they are and of what exactly they are to do."[65] Rather than defining pastoral theology clearly once and for all, Dykstra offers "a defiant embracing of" this insecurity and this madness, for there is a certain kind of freedom in being on the margins.

Dykstra offers in his edited volume nineteen different images of pastoral care—that is, nineteen different ways various pastoral theologians have tried to imagine what the field is. These images include the living human document (one by Anton Boisen and one by Charles Gerkin), the living human web (Bonnie Miller-McLemore), the solicitous shepherd (Seward Hiltner), the courageous shepherd (Alastair Campbell), the self-differentiated Samaritan (Jeanne Stevenson Moessner), the wounded healer (Henri Nouwen), the circus clown (Heije Faber), the wise fool (one by Alastair Campbell and one by Donald Capps), the intimate stranger (Robert Dykstra), the ascetic witness (James Dittes), the diagnostician (Paul Pruyser), the moral coach (Gaylord Noyce), the indigenous storyteller (Edward Wimberly), the agent of hope (Donald Capps), the midwife (Karen Hanson), the gardener (Margaret Zipse Kornfeld), and the midwife, storyteller, and reticent outlaw (Brita Gill-Austern).

Still, Dykstra *does* offer his own vision for the field, not just a collection of images. The fact that the field cannot be defined once and for all is indeed a part of his defining of the field. Other key features for Dykstra regarding the nature of pastoral theology, embedded in the introduction of *Images of Pastoral Care*, are the following five characteristics. First, *pastoral theologians work from the margins for the marginalized*. By this Dykstra means that, in seminary and other contexts, pastoral theologians rarely have the center stage or the place of honor. In theological seminaries, others (such as biblical scholars) often enjoy greater prestige (and higher salaries). In secular universities, pastoral theologians are rarely cited or even known by scholars in cognate fields (such as gender studies). By this—that is, working from the margins for the marginalized—Dykstra also means that pastoral theologians take special care in focusing their work on the marginalized of society, such as women, children, and other traditionally vulnerable persons and groups. Second, *pastoral theologians work with "psychology that matters."* Here, Dykstra means that pastoral theologians often privilege introspective and other experiential psychologies such as psychoanalytic psychologies (in contrast to empirical and behavioral psychologies) to do their work. Third, *the truths of pastoral theology are not universal; they are personal.* By this Dykstra means that, following Dittes, there is not a body of knowledge, as in, say, carpentry, that is being accumulated and passed down from one generation to the next because, when seeking knowledge about God or about human beings, nothing final can be known. The truth of pastoral theology is tested, verified, and refined by each generation and by each individual. Fourth, *pastoral theology is pluralistic and particularistic.* Other fields often try to find universals and generalities, knowledge of and for groups, but pastoral theology, as Dykstra envisions the field, has "a keen eye for the individual."[66] Pastoral theology, in other words, is local. Fifth, *the truths offered by pastoral theology are indirect and are often best captured by analogy and art such as poetry.* Since pastoral theology is concerned with emotion and with the human heart, the truths of pastoral theology, Dykstra suggests, cannot be reduced to logical maxims or scientific formulas. This point is especially important for this book.

Dykstra notes that the images offered in his book "function less as technical training guides or 'how-to' manuals for basic counseling or crisis intervention skills than . . . as works of art intent on inspiring ministry in more indirect and subtle ways."[67] Viewing pastoral images as evocative art, Dykstra notes three ways one may view art: (i) with *adoration*, as one (such as an Eastern Orthodox Christian) might view religious icons; (ii) with *disdain*, as one (such as a Protestant Christian) might view graven images/idols; and (iii) with *appreciation and critical appraisal*, as one (such as an art critic) might view works of art in museums. Dykstra endorses the third approach because it "seems to be the one that both honors the tradition and enables its adherents to adapt to new realities."[68]

An essay by Donald Capps explores this point made by Dykstra—that pastoral theology may be viewed as evocative art—in considerable detail, and in the following discussion I turn to it because I will use several insights from this essay as the basis for my own relating of pastoral theology and bioethics. Before that, however, some general discussion of correlational methodology is needed to ground this book in a wider intellectual schematic than pastoral theology, so that this book may be understood and appreciated as well as critiqued by a wider audience.

Paul Tillich's Method of Correlation

This book is an application of Paul Tillich's method of correlation. Tillich was born in Germany in 1886 and moved to the United States in 1933 after being denied a professorship by the Nazis. Because of his expansive mind, Tillich has been admired by many in various disciplines. Notably, Tillich has been of particular interest to pastoral theologians because, as Capps writes, he was "the one major theologian of the twentieth century who did not treat psychology—and psychologists—in a patronizing manner."[69]

Alister McGrath describes his method of correlation as "a conversation between human culture and Christian faith."[70] Reacting specifically against Karl Barth (another extremely influential theologian of the twentieth century), who, McGrath suggests, "attempted to drive a wedge between theology and culture," Tillich argued that "the gospel must speak to culture, and it can do so only if the actual questions raised by that culture are heard."[71] Thus, Tillich had a positive view of many so-called secular disciplines and fields, such as philosophy, psychology, psychoanalysis, literature, sociology, anthropology, the arts, and more, because these perspectives and tools are useful for gaining clarity regarding the questions raised by culture. McGrath adds that David Tracy (an important interpreter of Tillich) emphasizes that this dialogue between theology and culture "involves the mutual correction and enrichment of both gospel and culture."[72] In other words, it is insufficient to say that theology answers the questions raised by culture—the dialogue needs to go both ways.

Tillich explains his method in an essay titled "The Problem of Theological Method: II."[73] He writes:

> Question and answer must be correlated in such a way that the religious symbol is interpreted as the adequate answer to a question, implied in man's existence, and asked in primitive, pre-philosophical, or elaborated philosophical terms. For instance, the question implied in human finitude is answered in the symbols which constitute the idea of God . . . or the question implied in man's existential disruption and despair is answered in the symbol of Christ and his appearance under the conditions of existence. . . . The method of correlation establishes a mutual interdependence between questions and answers.[74]

For Tillich, theology is meaningful because it is existential.

In this book, my use of Tillich's method of correlation is idiosyncratic for at least two reasons. First, as one can see from Tillich's description of his method of correlation, he correlates major theological doctrines (such as the doctrine of the incarnation) with significant existential concerns (such as the experience of despair). Thus, as McGrath notes, Tillich is engaging in a form apologetics in that he is seeking to make contemporary theology relevant to and for a modern audience.[75] This is why Tillich has been referred to as an "apostle to the intellectuals."[76] In contrast, major theological doctrines are not a part of my correlations. Instead, I use images of pastoral care as sources of theology.

Second, I also am not taking central existential questions (such as, what is the meaning of human finitude?) as my focus for engaging culture. Rather, my focus is on core principles in bioethics. To be sure, while these principles do tend to raise grand questions about life and death, in my correlation of theology (i.e., influential images of pastoral care) and culture (i.e., core principles of bioethics), my intent is to uncover new—and sometimes mundane—issues for moral consideration.

Methodology and Art Theory

In this book, images of pastoral care and principles of bioethics are correlated, and this correlation is guided by art theory. In "The Lessons of Art Theory for Pastoral Theology," Capps explores possible relationships between theology and psychology in pastoral theology.[77] This point, as I will demonstrate in the following discussion, has implications for the relationship between principlist bioethics and pastoral theology.

While the relationship between theology and psychology in pastoral theology has generated a considerable body of literature, little of this literature views this relationship in light of art, which makes Capps's essay especially interesting. In this essay Capps reinvokes the term "perspective," a term that was widely used by the pioneers of pastoral theology,[78] by turning to various writings of art theorist Rudolf Arnheim.[79] Drawing on the insights of Arnheim, Capps proposes three models for the relationship between theology and psychology: convergence, juxtaposition, and structural uniformity. These three models are derived from three sets of observations by Capps about composition in the visual arts regarding (i) centric and eccentric forces, (ii) the problem of the divided center, and (iii) the depth dimension and the frontal plane. Capps's comments on centric and eccentric forces as well as the problem of the divided center are the features of his discussion that are most relevant for this book.

Capps notes, paraphrasing Arnheim, that centric forces are self-centered and that eccentric forces direct attention from the center to outer targets. "The centric tendency," Capps writes, "[of a] painting is usually located in or near the geometric center," and he also notes that "round and square paintings maximize the centric tendency, while rectangular paintings tend to de-emphasize it."[80] He points out that paintings featuring the Madonna with Child usually place Mary and Jesus at the center of the painting, thus emphasizing them. This is centricity. Often the center of the painting is the place of stability, the foundation on which everything is held together. An example of such a work is this icon of *Virgin and Child* (Figure 1.1). It is easy to see how this icon emphasizes Mary and Jesus by means of centricity.

The theoretical relevance for Capps regarding pastoral theology is that he identifies theology with centricity and psychology with eccentricity. So, to take this icon as a visual model for conceptualizing pastoral theology, the centric theological forces here could be viewed as emphasizing the divinity and the humanity of Jesus, while the eccentric psychological forces could be viewed as inviting reflection on the practical implications of the divinity and the humanity of Jesus both for the church and for the world, as the saints and the angels are looking away from the center. Thus, the value of psychology's eccentricity is that it can help to guard against theology's tendency to be self-centered, as when, for example, it has been said that during the middle ages theologians debated how many angels could fit (or dance) on the head of a needle (or pin). Such a debate is self-centered because it is difficult to imagine anyone outside of the Christian tradition caring about this debate. While this example may be extreme, debate about more mainstream doctrines,

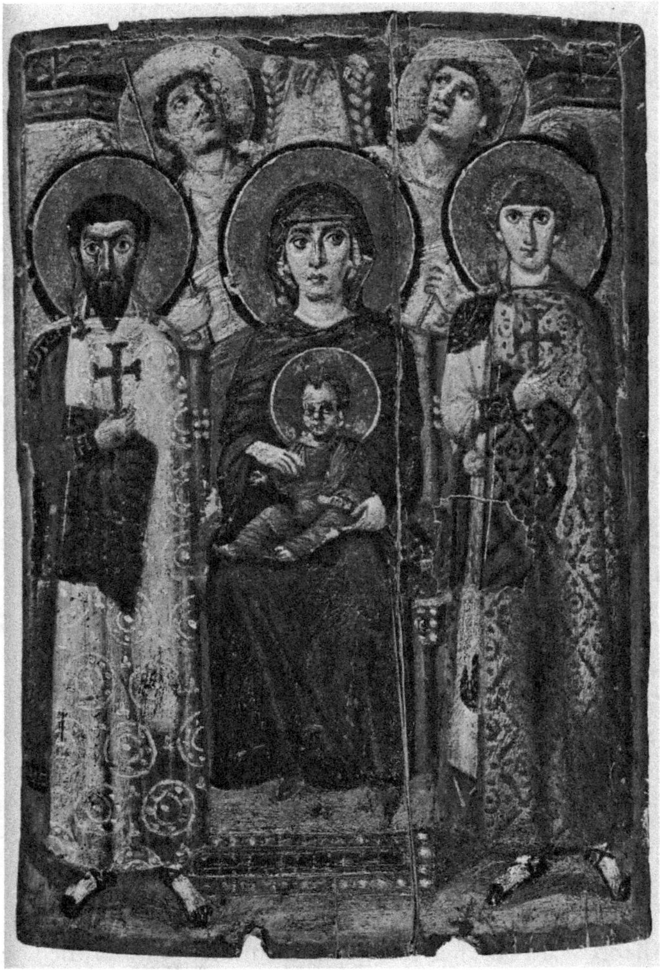

FIGURE 1.1. *Mary and Child* is an icon from the sixth century written by an unknown artist. It is in Saint Catherine's Monastery, Sinai, Egypt. This photograph, by K. Weitzmann, is a faithful reproduction of a work in the public domain. This work has been identified as being free of known restrictions under copyright law, including all related and neighboring rights: Public Domain Mark 1.0.

such as incarnation or atonement, also may appear to be insignificant to non-Christians.

Psychology helps theology to look beyond itself by making claims regarding human nature that are significant for non-Christians, such as teachings regarding spiritual formation and moral development. These teachings, which do draw on psychological findings, are of wider interest because they deal with perennial questions: *How does one become virtuous?*

In point of fact, drawing on theological education, medical educators have in recent years begun writing about professional identity formation, which is essentially spiritual formation in a secular context.[81]

Besides the possibility of centricity leading toward self-centeredness, Capps notes another complicating factor with regard to centricity, namely, that "the center can be the locus of tension." He cites Titian's *Noli Me Tangere* (Figure 1.2) as an example.

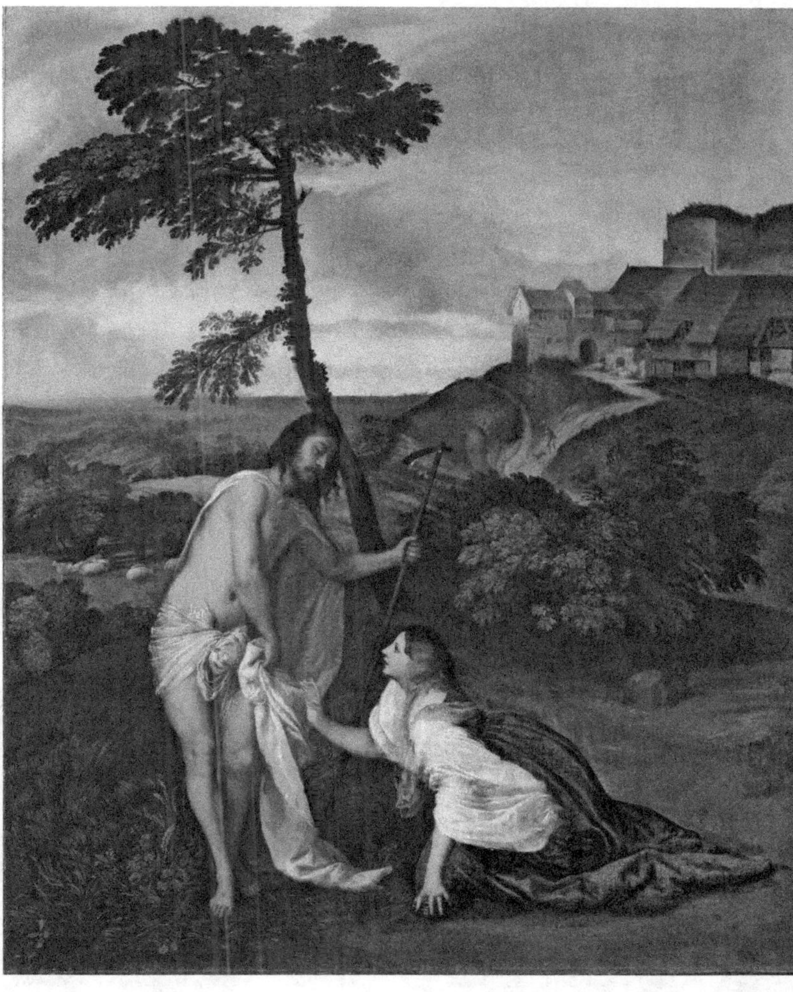

FIGURE 1.2. *Noli me tangere* is a *ca.* 1514 painting by Titian. It is in the collection of the National Gallery in London, United Kingdom. The source of the photograph is the National Gallery. This is a faithful reproduction of a work in the public domain. This work has been identified as being free of known restrictions under copyright law, including all related and neighboring rights: Public Domain Mark 1.0.

This painting depicts a scene after the resurrection of Jesus in which Jesus tells Mary Magdalene not to touch him (see John 20:17). In the painting there is a staff between Jesus and Mary, suggesting ambivalence (perhaps with regard to the ambiguous sexuality of Jesus[82]), Capps observes, thus imaging tension at the very center of this painting.

Similarly, with regard to the problem of the divided center, while sometimes the center can serve a stabilizing function (holding various aspects of a painting together), other times the center itself is divided (depicting perhaps even greater discord than ambivalence or tension), reflecting what Arnheim calls a bipolar composition. Capps writes: "This means that theology is not necessarily the calm at the center of the storm that rages around it, but is itself in conflict, the locus of controversy, struggle, and strife."[83] Capps suggests that Fra Angelico's *Annunciation* (Figure 1.3) is an artistic example of a divided center.

The central column achieves this division at the center quite effectively. This is a scene of controversy, struggle, and strife, as Mary contemplates the consequences of her pregnancy as an unwed woman, especially if her

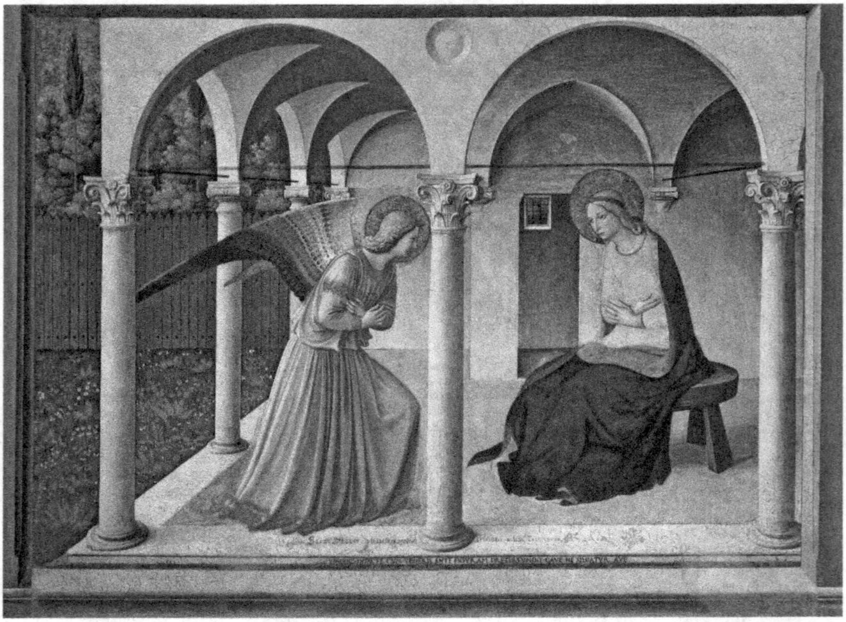

FIGURE 1.3. *The Annunciation* is a *ca.* 1438–45 fresco by Fra Angelico. It is in the Convent of San Marco in Florence, Italy. This is a faithful reproduction of a work in the public domain. This image is reproduced with permission by Bridgeman Images.

pregnancy were the result of a rape, perhaps by a Roman soldier, as some scholars have argued.[84]

How does this discussion pertain to the relationship between theology and psychology in pastoral theology? Capps explains:

> If we think of theology as representing the center and therefore as having a power that psychology, the eccentric and therefore more diffuse tendency, does not have, we should not assume that theology will necessarily act as the "balancing center" that stabilizes the picture overall. In fact, in paintings where the eccentric tendency is . . . marginalized . . . the tensions *within* the center are more likely to be enhanced. The dialogue, and the need for a bridging element, is not between representations of the centric and the eccentric forces within the painting, but between the figures who occupy the center. What this implies for pastoral theology is that the division *between* competing theological forces is as likely to require attention toward possible bridging as is the interaction between centric (theological) and eccentric (psychological) forces. This may also mean that the eccentric tendency will be the very element that enables the bipolarity of the center to be bridged.[85]

Capps adds: "I conclude from this that psychology . . . may well be the means whereby divisions created by conflicting *theological* viewpoints of pastoral theologians may be mediated, even reconciled."[86]

A Pastoral Aesthetic for Bioethics

My suggestion, informed by Capps's discussion of art theory, is that *the four principles of bioethics may be viewed as centric forces* in bioethics and that *pastoral theology may be viewed as an eccentric force*. To be clear, when I use the term "eccentric," I do not mean strange or odd. Rather, I mean looking *at* or *from* the margins. Also, perhaps sometimes pastoral theology may be able to serve as a bridging element in bioethics, between, say, competing understandings of justice, but that is not my primary objective in this book. My concern is to demonstrate that pastoral theology can draw attention to a variety of margins, not unlike the serene imagery of Titian's *Noli Me Tangere* on the margins of the painting. The center is not the only thing worth looking at.

By envisioning pastoral theology as aesthetic imagination, Dykstra emphasizes that he is not offering a how-to manual with regard to the practice of pastoral care but rather a sensibility of and for pastoral theology, a sensibility that is akin to critical art appreciation. This book does the same for bioethics, for it, too, is not a how-to manual. It offers a way of looking at things.

The next four chapters of this book examine one of the four principles of bioethics, so, in this sense, they are centric forces. But in each chapter the principle also will be viewed through the lens of an image of pastoral care; the image of pastoral care will serve as an eccentric force. In doing so, each chapter will offer:

- a discussion of the bioethics principle,
- an illustration or two of the principle,
- a discussion of the image of pastoral care, and
- a correlation of the principle and the image.

In each case, the analysis will be theologically-informed, psychologically-sophisticated, therapeutically-oriented, and experientially-grounded, though chapter 5 will be slightly different in this regard, for reasons that will become obvious later.

A Precursor

I would be remiss if I did not draw attention to an important precursor to this book: William May's *The Physician's Covenant: Images of the Healer in Medical Ethics*.[87] May suggests that ethics provides a kind of "corrective vision."[88] He writes:

> Ethics supplies a type of *corrective* lens. Ethics relies heavily on the distinction between what is and what ought to be. Such corrective vision, however, challenges not so much the world the descriptive sciences see as the world distorted through the bias of institutional structures or through the prism of human imperfection and vice.[89]

"We cannot change our behavior," May adds, "unless, in some respects, our perception of the world also changes."[90] The task of the ethicist, in other words, is to offer new perspectives on moral problems. Sometimes this means helping to resolve dilemmas, but not always. May focuses on images in his book, and he does so because images help us to perceive and also to express what we have perceived. "An image," he writes, "tells a kind of compressed story, not a particular story about an identifiable person, not an exemplary story designed to inspire, but a prototypical story to which all specific narratives bear a kind of family resemblance."[91]

Some images shape and order our experience. In bioethics circles, the four principles of respect for autonomy, beneficence, nonmaleficence, and justice have taken on, as it were, iconic status, shaping and ordering bioethics discourse. Yet what May offers is in tension with, or at least different from, mainstream bioethics:

> As a guide to practice, images function differently from moral principles and they imply somewhat different views of the moral agent. Philosophical ethics, as usually taught, orients less to image than to principles; it presupposes not the ordinary volume of work with which the practitioner must cope but the exceptional case. It assumes that the practitioner is riddled with uncertainty in facing a particular decision and seeks help from the ethicist in identifying the right set of principles to resolve the quandary.[92]

What May offers is this:

> Images do not function quite so successfully in those situations which the moralists call hard cases. They do not operate as a manual for getting the decision maker out of an exceptional moral bind in which he or she does not know what to do. Rather, they provide a comprehensive ordering of life—an interpretation of role, metaphysical setting, and institutional context—that makes moral behavior seem more like a rite repeated than a puzzle solved. An image provides a compelling picture of the world and one's role in it.[93]

The images of doctors that May focuses on include parent, fighter, technician, and teacher. Each of these images, he argues, has strengths and weaknesses, and each offer its own moral vision of medicine, but the image that May argues for is the physician as one who makes a covenant. While I do not offer or advocate for a particular image to guide medicine and/or bioethics, my goal, inspired by May, is to stimulate new ways of perceiving in bioethics.

2 RESPECT FOR AUTONOMY AND THE LIVING HUMAN DOCUMENT

I asked Jon Wolfshohl, an emergency room physician, about how he understands that the principle of respect for autonomy is relevant to the lives of practicing clinicians. He replied: "coding."[1]

In the United States, many older adults die in hospitals, more so today than in the past, when it was more common to die at home.[2] Technology—which can support the lungs, provide artificial nutrition and hydration, and more—has made it possible to delay death in ways that were not imaginable one hundred years ago. However, the quality-of-life resulting is sometimes not desirable to some patients (more on this in chapter 3), in part because the means of delaying death entails coding. Coding involves aggressive techniques such as cardiopulmonary resuscitation (CPR) that include chest compressions, which routinely and unintentionally break the ribs of elderly patients. After this, such patients then are connected to many machines, sometimes until they die, perhaps days or weeks or months later. This is painful for everyone involved—patients, families, and caregivers.

To prevent this scenario from playing out, medical teams present patients and families with the option of signing a do-not-resuscitate (DNR) order so that patients may be allowed to die without aggressive interference from medical teams. These conversations can be difficult for many reasons, including a reluctance to accept dying as well as an inaccurate understanding of what coding entails. For Wolfshohl, respect for autonomy is especially relevant to coding because, if patients or families do not understand the implications of their decisions in a concrete way, it is unclear if autonomy has been actually respected: "Do they really want *this*?" Wolfshohl wonders.

Though illegal, some clinicians disobey the wishes of patients and families who request that everything be done by means of "slow coding" or "no coding" (acting like one is trying to save the life of a patient but is instead faking the chest compressions or carrying out procedures slowly on purpose, so as to hasten death[3]). To be sure, Wolfshohl is not advocating slow coding or no coding. Rather, he is identifying a key area where respecting patient autonomy is difficult in practice, both for him and for many clinicians.

Upon further reflection, Wolfshohl also told me that when people present to the emergency department, patients are often "not themselves." He continued: "Sometimes they obviously do not have decision-making capacity, if they are unconscious or if they are in the midst of a psychotic episode, but other times the way in which patients are not themselves is more subtle—for example, after a traumatic event. People just are not thinking clearly, for understandable reasons." Wolfshohl explained to me that his goals are, first, to address acute problems that may cause death and, second, to help patients get in touch with what he calls their "true self." "Because patients are emotionally unraveled when they present to the emergency department," he told me, "I want to find ways to empower patients so that they can have some sense of control over their lives, which I think of as autonomy."[4]

In talking with Wolfshohl about how he attempts to empower patients, he told me that one strategy that he has adopted is from a case he read about in *Living in Limbo: Life in the Midst of Uncertainty*.[5] The case is by Tapani Ahola, a social psychologist.[6] Siru, a fifteen-year-old girl, was an inpatient at a psychiatric hospital, and after a few months, Ahola was asked to provide an assessment of her progress. Siru seemed to be doing well. In interviewing her, Siru explained that her father had committed suicide and that this became overwhelming for her. One of the nurses, who was present during this interview, interjected and added that Siru's father had suffered from alcoholism. They talked for a considerable amount of time about the many problems and difficulties in Siru's life. Near the conclusion of the interview, Ahola said to Siru:

> You have gone through a very rough period in your life, and what has happened has had a great impact on you. It may be impossible for you to foresee what the effects will be in the long run, but let's imagine sometime in the distant future you are a grandmother with an adult daughter and a teenage granddaughter. You have told your daughter about your father's suicide and about the time you spent in a mental hospital. Your daughter, in turn, has told your story to her daughter. Your story will serve as a teaching story. It will be wisdom that is of

> value not only to your daughter but also to your granddaughter. What do you imagine that wisdom might be?[7]

Siru's wisdom was this: "First, I've realized that it is possible to survive even the most terrible things," and, "second, I used to be the kind of person who kept my thoughts to myself. That wasn't good. Here at the hospital I've learned that talking helps."[8] Ahola, then, closed this interview by focusing on her progress (not her problems), and this helped Siru to cultivate hope in her life and to adopt practical strategies that work for her.

Wolfshohl, as noted, modified Ahola's approach for the context of emergency medicine, a context that is very different from the context of a psychiatric hospital. Wolfshohl deals with acute crises that, after addressed, often result in a patient being transferred to another department. He sees patients after accidents, suicide attempts, strokes, rapes, and cardiac events, to list just some of the common scenarios. Also, Wolfshohl's time with patients is limited. Further, in many cases he never sees a particular patient again. Despite all of these differences, Wolfshohl explained to me what he took away from Ahola's case. After attending to a patient's presenting problem, he will say some version of the following:

> I understand that you are in crisis. We are going to take care of you. And while I need to attend to another patient briefly, I will be back shortly. In the meantime, I want you to do one thing for me: Think about your future self, sometime when this crisis is in the distant past—maybe 10 years. What advice would your future self give you about your situation now? I'd like to hear this advice when I return. Can you do that for me?[9]

In almost every case, this turns out to be a positive exercise. Like Siru, Wolfshohl's patients begin to find some hope in their current situation. The value of this approach, Wolfshohl has found, is that it creates possibilities for healing when he is not in the room. He added: "It also gives me a sense I can trust more fully the decisions that these patients are making, because they are calmer. I realize that I do not know them, but they really do seem more like themselves, perhaps in part because they have claimed some autonomy in a situation in which they feel powerless."

Part One: The Principle

The focus of this chapter is on respect for autonomy.[10] In part one, I begin by providing an overview of the principle and then review a classic case in bioethics (the case of Karen Ann Quinlan). This illustrates how the principle is often understood. Next, in part two, I move to a discussion of Anton Boisen's pastoral image of the living human document. The essential feature of this image is that it provides a theological rationale for studying human experience, especially the ways in which persons can experience their lives as disorganized when confronted with illness (e.g., when patients present to the psychiatric hospital or the emergency department). In part three I correlate respect for autonomy and the living human document by focusing on the novel *A Monster Calls*, using Sigmund Freud's theory of dreams to interpret a key scene from the story. The central claim of this chapter is that a pastoral perspective on respect for autonomy can shift the focus away from respecting choices to appreciating individuals and that this shift facilitates the potential to improve caregiving.

In making this argument, I use psychoanalysis to interpret literature. Other schools of psychology will be used elsewhere in this book. Also, while I use a novel to explore experience, other means of inquiry, such as memoirs, could be used as well. Indeed, other expressions of experience will be used in this book. The key point is that there is much to be gained by understanding patients as living human documents.

Respect for Autonomy

While Beauchamp and Childress begin their list of principles with respect for autonomy, they are quick to point out that this should not imply that this principle has more weight than other principles—the most common criticism of their work, as noted previously. They also note that others have criticized their work as individualistic, reason-centric, and legalistic. They deny these characterizations.

Beauchamp and Childress point out that the term "autonomy" is derived from Greek, meaning "self-rule." "At a minimum," they write, "personal autonomy encompasses self-rule that is free from both controlling interference by others and limitations that prevent meaningful choice, such as inadequate understanding,"[11] due to, for example, dementia, psychosis, and so on. Two conditions are key for them for autonomy to be realized: liberty (being free from control) and agency (being free to act).

Beauchamp and Childress assert three necessary conditions for autonomous choice: intention, understanding, and noncoercion. With regard to patient care they offer these rules as specifications of respect for autonomy: (i) tell the truth; (ii) respect the privacy of others; (iii) protect confidential information; (iv) obtain consent for interventions; and (v) help others make important decisions when asked to do so.

It is important to point out that telling the truth is at the top of their list of rules. While it may seem noncontroversial to suggest that patients should be told the truth about their diagnosis and prognosis, in the 1970s it was common for patients not to be told everything about a cancer diagnosis because it was believed patients would become depressed and lose hope as well as the will to live.[12] Today the issue is a little different, though no less important, as when patients from various cultural contexts (e.g., Eastern Europe, Asia) do not want to know if they have a terminal illness.[13] The current thinking among western countries is that asking patients if they want to know their diagnosis is a way of respecting their autonomy—that, in other words, information should not be forced on patients. Relatedly, sometimes clinicians mislead patients by using specialized language (words like carcinoma instead of cancer)[14] or by being less than forthright regarding prognosis.[15] These are examples of *not* respecting the autonomy of patients.

Beauchamp and Childress offer an interesting discussion in this regard concerning a research study that focused on Navajo values. Its purpose was to determine how to provide culturally competent patient care to this demographic. In traditional Navajo culture, it is believed that "thought and language have the power to shape reality and to control events."[16] Beauchamp and Childress write: "According to the traditional conception, telling a Navajo patient recently diagnosed with a disease the potential complications of that disease may actually produce those complications, because 'language does not merely describe reality, language shapes reality.' "[17] Thus, revealing prognostic information may actually be, in certain circumstances, a violation of respect for autonomy.

Beauchamp and Childress again emphasize that respect for autonomy often entails consent, but they add that consent is neither always necessary nor always sufficient in the final analysis because during public health emergencies autonomy can be overruled in favor of other communal considerations regarding public safety (e.g., federal law in the United States requires people to undergo certain treatments if infected with tuberculosis). They also note a variety of forms of consent: explicit, implicit, and presumed. Explicit consent (or informed consent) receives the most attention in bioethics literature.

It rose to prominence during the decades following World War II after the Nuremberg trials, by which Nazi doctors and others were tried for conducing horrific experiments on various groups of human beings, most notably Jewish persons. But other forms of consent are equally important. Implicit consent, for example, is when patients come to a teaching hospital for treatment. Simply by showing up they consent to many different health professionals—for example, nurses and doctors—at varying levels of training to treat them. Yet some controversy remains, however, such as when eight or more medical students, interns, and residents practice pelvic and/or rectal exams on anesthetized patients without explicit consent.[18] Presumed consent is a form of implied consent based on what is known about a person from previous conversations and interactions.

A complication relating to consent is that patients sometimes change their minds. Which preference holds more weight? Beauchamp and Childress suggest that it is helpful to inquire whether a given choice seems in-character or out-of-character. Still, there is obviously room for disagreement in this regard. Beauchamp and Childress note a case of a twenty-eight-year-old man who decided to terminate his kidney dialysis because his quality-of-life was very poor. He said to the clinical staff that, even if he requested to be put back on dialysis while he was dying, not to do so, because he feared that he would change his mind while in pain. He did. But his team did not put him back on dialysis, and he died. Was his autonomy respected in this case? It is not obvious.

Another key concept for Beauchamp and Childress is competence. They define competence as "the ability to perform a task."[19] Because tasks vary, the criteria for particular competencies vary, meaning that competence can change over time or it can come and go (as with cases of acute psychosis). In medical contexts competence usually centers on whether a patient can understand a procedure, assess its risks and benefits, and make a decision.

Informed consent is a topic in bioethics closely related to competence. Beauchamp and Childress note that in bioethics literature there are two meanings of informed consent—individual and institutional. An individual's informed consent means that they are authorizing a specific medical intervention or deciding to participate in a research study, while informed consent with regard to an institution means satisfying a procedural process, usually involving the signing of paperwork. Beauchamp and Childress offer these seven elements of informed consent:

1. competence,
2. voluntariness,

3. disclosure of clinical and/or research information,
4. recommendation of a plan,
5. understanding of disclosure and proposed plan,
6. decision, and
7. authorization.

Noting that there is some ambiguity as to what ought to be disclosed—not all medical information can be conveyed to patients—they discuss special cases of intentional nondisclosure such as cases of therapeutic privilege (e.g., when patients are too agitated to hear certain information) and therapeutic use of placebos (e.g., prescription of an antibiotic for a common cold).

Beauchamp and Childress also note that there is ambiguity about understanding. There are many common terms among health professionals—for example, stoke and hernia—that patients may not understand. This applies to research, too. Beauchamp and Childress cite a striking study where 90% of research participants enrolled in a cancer clinical trial indicated that they were "well informed" about the trial but "approximately three-fourths of them did not understand that the trial included nonstandard and unproven treatment, and approximately one-fourth did not appreciate that the primary purpose of the trial was to benefit future patients and that the benefits to them personally were uncertain."[20] Still other complicating factors with regard to informed consent include the signing of waivers (e.g., when patients request not to be informed of risks during surgery) and when patients hold false beliefs or beliefs inconsistent with science (e.g., believing that one does not have cancer when biopsy results are conclusive in this regard).

In concluding the chapter, Beauchamp and Childress note that "the intimate connection between autonomy and decision-making in health care and research, especially in circumstances of consent and refusal, unifies this chapter's several sections."[21] Indeed, virtually all of their chapter focuses on decision-making—with disclosure, competence, and informed consent being the key topics—in one way or another. But they also note that respect for autonomy remains open to interpretation, thus inviting more reflection on the principle.

An Illustration: The Case of Karen Ann Quinlan

Respect for autonomy in patient care and clinical research focuses on, for Beauchamp and Childress, choice. Given that there are many situations in medicine when patients cannot make decisions and also that some of these situations are created or exacerbated by developments in medical technology, bioethics as a field has had a major focus on, not surprisingly, comas and other such states where choice becomes equivocal, where it is difficult to know what a patient in impaired states (such as psychosis or depression) really wants or would want or what to do when surrogates such as family members disagree.

One of the earliest cases that helped to launch the field of bioethics is the case of Karen Ann Quinlan. Gregory Pence discusses this case in *Classic Cases in Medical Ethics: Accounts of Cases that Have Shaped Medical Ethics, with Philosophical, Legal, and Historical Backgrounds.*[22] He notes that in 1975 Quinlan, who was then twenty-one years old, was found unresponsive in her bed after a night of drinking with her friends. They called an ambulance for help. Though she was revived, she never regained consciousness. Medical technology kept her alive.

Pence notes that a bottle of Valium was found in her purse, and blood tests revealed that Quinlan had been taking benzodiazepines or barbiturates (or both), mixed with alcohol. The court records are unclear on this point. She appeared to be dieting or fasting as well, as she only weighed 115 pounds. This also could have been a factor in her unresponsiveness. As it turned out, Quinlan had entered a persistent vegetative state (PVS), meaning that, while she was not braindead, she was not conscious either. Also, Quinlan presented with periods of wakefulness, which is unlike a coma. Her sister described it this way:

> Whenever I thought of a person in a coma, I thought they would just lie there very quietly, almost as though they were sleeping. Karen's head was moving around, as if she was trying to pull away from that tube in her throat, and she made little noises, like moans. I don't know if she was in pain, but it seemed as though she was. And I thought—if Karen could ever see herself like this, it would be the worst thing in the world for her.[23]

A lawyer gave this description:

> Her eyes are open and move in a circular manner as she breathes; her eyes blink approximately three or four times per minute; her forehead evidences very noticeable perspiration; her mouth is open while the respirator expands to ingest oxygen, and while her mouth is open, her tongue appears to be moving in a rather random manner; her mouth closes as the oxygen is ingested into her body through the tracheotomy

> and she appears to be slightly convulsing or gasping as the oxygen enters her windpipe; her hands are visible in an emaciated form, facing in a praying position away from her body. Her present weight would seem to be in the vicinity of 70–80 pounds.[24]

Pence notes that the hospital gave her a one-in-a-million chance of recovering, and, after a few months, the Quinlan family agreed that the respirator should be withdrawn, allowing Quinlan to die. Pence adds that according to Roman Catholic teaching (the family's religious heritage) respirators are considered extraordinary treatment and therefore may be withheld or withdrawn.

But after the family agreed to withdraw the respirator, the physicians attending to Quinlan refused to do so, fearing a malpractice lawsuit. The Quinlan family therefore took their case to court. After a number of appeals, the New Jersey Supreme Court ruled in favor of the Quinlan family, instructing that the respirator should be withdrawn. Then, instead of simply disconnecting the respirator, the physicians attending to Quinlan weaned her off slowly. Eventually Quinlan was able to breathe without the respirator. Pence writes, "This weaning created some confusion in the general public: Some people took it to mean that Karen had gotten better; others took it to mean that Karen's physicians 'had pulled the plug' and that a miracle must have occurred because she hadn't died—but both impressions were false."[25] Quinlan lived for another ten years, never regaining consciousness. She died after contracting pneumonia. Of note, the Quinlan family declined antibiotics that would have treated the pneumonia.

This case fits with respect for autonomy because it was not clear then who should have made decisions for Quinlan when she was unable to do so for herself. But the case raises many other issues in bioethics: Should life be preserved at all costs? What criteria should be used to determine death? To what extent should prognosis factor into treatment decisions? Are there moral differences between withdrawing and withholding treatment, between extraordinary and ordinary care?

Part Two: The Image

Having provided an overview of respect for autonomy, as well as an illustration of it, I now want to turn to the living human document to set the stage for offering a pastoral perspective on respect for autonomy.

The Living Human Document

As noted in chapter 1, Boisen is often regarded as the founder of the clinical pastoral education (CPE) movement, and he may be regarded as the father of modern pastoral theology as well. Once an inpatient in a psychiatric hospital on account of his delusions and hallucinations, Boisen lived after this hospitalization in psychiatric hospitals his whole life, sometimes as a chaplain and other times, during relapses, as a patient.[26] Robert Dykstra writes:

> In those initial months of hospitalization Boisen discovered what from that point on would become his singular calling. His own unsettling experiences convinced him that the emotional breakdowns psychiatric patients suffered were often religious in origin. Therefore, he reasoned, they could not be effectively treated without taking religious and philosophical concerns into account.[27]

Dykstra notes that Boisen then began working on a way to bring ministry into the clinical setting, and he eventually did so by bringing seminary students into psychiatric hospitals on the grounds that seminary students should study what he called "human documents."[28] His main thesis was that seminary students should study not only sacred texts, such as the Bible and religious creeds, but also the lived experiences of persons. Boisen describes his early efforts as follows:

> In the summer of 1925 I was given the opportunity to try the experiment of bringing some theological students to the hospital. These students worked on the wards as ordinary attendants. My own experience had convinced me that there is no one upon whom the patient's welfare is more dependent than the nurse or attendant who is with him hour after hour during the day. I felt also that such work provided an unequaled opportunity to observe and understand the patient, and I was much concerned that theological students should have the opportunity to go to first-hand sources for their knowledge of human nature. I wanted them to learn to read human documents as well as books.[29]

Thus, living human documents refers to the experiences of persons, especially patients.

Reflecting on his image of the living human document, Boisen writes: "I had at this time [of writing] done no reading whatever in psychiatric literature . . . [so] the conclusions were drawn entirely from my own experience and observations in light of the work I had previously done in the psychology of religion."[30] He continues:

> I see two main cases of insanity. In one case there is some organic trouble, a defect in the brain tissue . . . . In the other there is no organic difficulty. The body is strong, and the brain in good working order. The difficulty is rather in the *disorganization of the patient's world*. Something has happened which has upset the foundations upon which his ordinary reasoning is based. Death or disappointment or sense of failure may have compelled a reconstruction of the patient's worldview from the bottom up, and the mind becomes dominated by the one idea which he has been trying to put in its proper place.[31]

Thus, Boisen has a special interest in how persons can experience their lives as disorganized.

In some strands of theology (especially liberal protestant theology), human experience is regarded as inherently theological because human experience is believed to be a source of revelation from God, in addition to other sources such as scripture. This claim has been key for pastoral theology due, in no small way, to Boisen's work.

But what does it mean to take human experience seriously, to regard human experience as a source of revelation? In *Lament for a Son*, Nicholas Wolterstorff, who taught philosophical theology at Yale University, writes about his experience of grief after the sudden death of his son, who died in a climbing accident. He writes: "For a long time I knew that God is not the impassive, unresponsive, unchanging being portrayed by the classical theologians. . . . God is not only the God of sufferers but the God who suffers. The pain and fallenness of humanity have entered into his heart. Through the prism of my tears I have seen a suffering God."[32] For Wolterstorff, God became more fully known through his experience of grief, and he concluded that the classical theologians were wrong: God suffers. This theological insight was revealed to Wolterstorff via experience.

Other schools of theology make similar claims. For example, in *The Cross and the Lynching Tree*, James Cone explores the meaning of the Gospel in light of various experiences of oppression—especially murder—of African Americans in the United States.[33] Relatedly, much of holocaust and postholocaust theology is dedicated to making sense of God and tradition in light of the experiences of Jewish people and others who suffered during and after World War II.[34] Thus, whether focusing on the experiences of individuals (like Wolterstorff) or communities (such as African Americans), taking human experience seriously means that we know God, in part, by knowing ourselves and by listening to others. That is to say, knowing God is accomplished not only by prayerfully studying canonical sacred texts but also by judiciously attending to living human documents.

Part Three: Correlation of Principle and Image

In correlating respect for autonomy and the living human document, I turn to *A Monster Calls*,[35] an award-winning novel by Patrick Ness about thirteen-year-old Conor O'Malley whose mother is dying of cancer. In doing so, I treat Conor as a living human document.[36]

I realize that using a novel about the family member of a patient who has cancer (rather than a novel about a patient who has cancer) might seem to be an odd choice in discussing respect for autonomy, but such a move actually enables me to write about this principle in a new way. In what follows I explore what Boisen describes as the disorganization of the patient's world in the life of Conor through the lens of psychoanalysis.

As detailed in chapter 1, a major critique of principlist bioethics is that it tends to offer decontextualized (i.e., thin) accounts of moral experience. In *Bioethics, Culture, and Identity: A Philosophical Disease*, Carl Elliott also makes this point and notes that novels are one way that accounts of moral experience can be thickened for a very simple reason: fiction writers "are better at telling stories than philosophers, lawyers, and doctors."[37] Relatedly, in *Narrative Medicine: Honoring the Stories of Illness*, Rita Charon critiqued the common practice in medical schools of assigning short stories: "Hugh Crawford cautioned us years ago [that] the conventional restriction . . . to the genre of the short story limits the work we are able to do with students," and adds, "students need the experience of living with a narrator through a long work of fiction as well as the short form."[38] In medical schools, since the required curriculum is extremely full, the time allotted to medical humanities (as well as ethics, professionalism, etc.) is necessarily limited, and, not surprisingly, medical educators have relied on short stories (instead of novels) for pragmatic reasons. Be that as it may, if many critics of mainstream bioethics argue that more attention to context and to experience is needed (a critique with which Crawford and Charon would agree), my use of a novel in this chapter is meant to respond to such critiques.

As an example of a thin case study that is typical in bioethics texts, Elliott offers the following: "A child is born prematurely and suffers anoxic brain damage. He is currently on a ventilator and if he survives he will always be profoundly mentally retarded. Should treatment be discontinued?"[39]

If the case of Conor explored in this chapter were written in this genre, it could be summed up as follows: "A thirteen-year-old boy, whose parents are divorced, is experiencing deep feelings of ambivalence (expressed in nightmares) in response to his mother dying. He is demonstrating asocial behavior at school. Should the boy be referred to a health professional, such as a psychiatrist or a social worker?" While this vignette may be accurate, and also while the question is a legitimate one, the depth of Conor's ambivalence cannot be conveyed by these few lines. More is needed to attend to Conor as a living human document. Thus, this chapter is an endorsement of those who affirm the usefulness of fiction for bioethics.

The Case of Conor O'Malley

The following is a brief synopsis of the book, intended to set up a critical reading of the narrative through the lens of dream theory. Because this synopsis is necessarily brief, I hope it encourages readers to buy *A Monster Calls*, particularly the illustrated version, as the writing of Patrick Ness (the author) and the illustrations by Jim Kay (the artist) are remarkably beautiful and emotionally moving.

A Monster Calls, set in present-day England, begins with a yew tree monster appearing after midnight, apparently in a dream, to visit thirteen-year-old Conor O'Malley. Conor has been experiencing a recurring nightmare that involves his mother falling over a cliff after being pulled over by a different monster. Throughout much of the book, it is not clear as to whether the yew tree monster is real, a dream, or something else. But what is clear is that it showed up around the time his mother was dying of cancer. In any case, during one visit to Conor the yew tree monster explained to Conor that he would tell him three stories and that, after he has finished, Conor would be required to tell him a fourth story—about Conor's personal truth. While Conor was not afraid of the yew tree monster, the idea of telling his personal truth terrified him.

Conor's grandmother came to visit. She told him that his mother was going back to the hospital because the treatment was not working. She added that his father would be visiting, all the way from the United States, which greatly surprised him because Conor's parents were divorced. Later, Conor asked his mother why she was going back to the hospital. She told him that she was going to be okay. But Conor pressed her, wanting the truth. She just hugged him.

At his grandma's house Conor didn't feel welcome because it was very clean and filled with antiques. When his father arrived, Conor said that he would like to live with his father in the United States, that he did not want to live with his grandmother, but his father said that there was no room for him there (he remarried and had a new child), though he did invite Conor to visit at Christmas.

Sometime later Conor was in his grandmother's house alone. He looked at the clock, touched it, and realized he had broken it by accident. The yew tree monster, somehow able to be in the room with him, said that he had come to tell him a tale, and he transported Conor to 150 years ago. Conor thought he was dreaming. This tale ended with the yew tree monster destroying a house in the dream, and Conor joined in, but when Conor awoke he discovered that he was in his grandmother's house and that he had destroyed her sitting room. The yew tree monster was nowhere to be found. Conor had destroyed so many of his grandmother's precious belongings and he didn't understand what had happened, for there was too much destruction for this to have been done by him alone. Just then his grandmother returned home, and when she saw the mess, she groaned and screamed and then went to her room and wept. Conor tried to clean up the mess, but there was too much for him to do so.

The next day when Conor came down for breakfast he found that his father had come over because Conor's grandmother called him early in the morning on account of Conor's mother getting worse. Conor's father did not discipline him for destroying the room and said that they were going to ignore this because of Conor's mother's health. Conor seemed disappointed that he wasn't going to be punished.

At school everyone kept their distance. He didn't turn in his homework, and his teachers let this slide. No one was punishing Conor for anything. After school Conor went to see his mother. She explained that the treatments weren't working but that there was one more treatment that they were going to try: *one made from a yew tree*. Conor's thoughts began to race. Is *this*, he wondered, why the yew tree monster came to visit him—to save his mother? Conor was cautiously hopeful.

Days passed. His grandmother would not talk to him. No one at school would talk with him. His mother was too tired to talk, and his father had nothing to say on the phone. Even the yew tree monster stopped visiting.

Later, Conor was taken from class to the hospital. He never had been taken from school before, so Conor was afraid. When he went into his mother's room, she was sitting up, looking as though she was getting better. The yew tree worked, he thought! But then he saw his mother's eyes. She was sad. She told him that the treatment from the yew tree wasn't working. Conor asked what the next treatment was, but she replied that there would be no more treatments. Angry, Conor accused his mother of lying. She replied: "I think, deep in your heart, you've always known," and she added, "It's okay that you're angry, sweetheart," and "You be as angry as you need to be. . . . Don't let anyone tell you otherwise. Not your grandma, not your dad, no one. And if you need to break things, then by God, you break them good and hard."[40] She continued: "And if, one day . . . you look back and you feel bad for being so angry, if you feel bad for being *so* angry at me that you couldn't even speak to me, then you have to know, Conor, you have to know that it was *okay*. It was okay. That I *knew*. I *know*, okay? I know everything you need to tell me without you having to say it out loud. All right?"[41] Conor nodded.

Conor demanded to go back to his house, and his grandmother complied. Conor made his way to the tree. He called to it and then kicked it. Nothing happened. But then the yew tree monster appeared. Conor wanted to know why he came, if not to heal his mother.

The yew tree monster replied that Conor was the one who called him. Conor, breaking down, asked for the yew tree monster to help him. The yew tree monster replied that it was time for Conor to tell the fourth tale.

Conor found himself in a dark forest near a cliff. His mother was farther ahead of him, dangerously close to the edge. She looked back to Conor and smiled but looked weak. Conor yelled for her to get away from the cliff but she didn't move. Conor ran to her. Conor heard a noise from over the cliff. It was a monster—the *real* monster, not the yew tree monster—though he knew he couldn't get there in time. Two giant hands from over the cliff grabbed her and began pulling her over. Conor ran and, just in time, grabbed her hands. This is where Conor's nightmare always began.

His mother yelled for Conor not to let go. The nightmare monster pulled harder. She began to slip from Conor's hands. Conor looked back at the yew tree monster, asking for help, but he did nothing. She slipped more, and Conor grew weak. The yew tree monster demanded that Conor speak the truth. Conor refused. His mother fell.

While Conor usually woke up at this point in the nightmare, this time he did not, and he stood there with the yew tree monster. He repeated that Conor still needed to speak the truth. But Conor told the yew tree monster to take him out of here so that he could see his mother. The yew tree monster said that she is no longer here, that he—Conor—let her go. Conor objected, saying that she fell. But the yew tree monster would not relent: he demanded that Conor admit that he let her go. The yew tree monster demanded that Conor speak the truth, but Conor said that he didn't know it.

Then Conor realized that he *did* know the truth. The yew tree monster again asked him to speak the truth, this time in a kind tone. Conor began to cry. And he asked the yew tree monster not to make him say it. The yew tree monster said that Conor *wanted* her to fall. Conor yelled "No!" The yew tree monster demanded that he speak the truth, but Conor again refused. He demanded to know *why* Conor let his mother go. Then Conor spoke the truth: "I can't stand knowing that she'll go! I just want it to be over! I want it to be *finished*!"[42]

When Conor awoke from the nightmare he felt as though he deserved death. The yew tree monster was still there. Conor said to him that he did indeed know that his mother was not going to live, but he wanted to believe that she could, though the waiting was just terrible. Conor began crying, heavily. The yew tree monster said: "*And a part of you wished it would just end . . . even if it meant losing her.*"[43] Conor nodded. But Conor added, "I didn't *mean* it, though. . . . I didn't mean to let her go! And now it's for real! Now she's going to die and it's my fault!"[44] "*And that*, the yew tree monster said, "*is not the truth at all.*"[45] The yew tree monster reassured Conor by telling him that wishing for pain to end is very human. Conor said that he didn't mean it, but the yew tree monster said that he did mean it and also that he didn't mean it as well. Conor wondered how both could be true. The yew tree monster replied, "*Because humans are complicated beasts*," and added:

> *Your mind will contradict itself a hundred times each day. You wanted her to go at the same time you were desperate for me to save her. Your mind will believe comforting lies while also knowing the painful truths that make those lies necessary. And your mind will punish you for believing both.*[46]

Conor wanted to know how to fight these competing forces, and the yew tree monster said by speaking the truth about oneself. He added that it is not important what one *thinks* but rather what one *does*. Conor then asked the yew tree monster what he should do. The yew tree monster told him to speak the truth. Exhausted, Conor fell asleep.

Conor awoke to his grandmother's voice, and she rushed him back to the hospital. When they arrived, they found Conor's mother, sleeping. Conor's grandmother grabbed her hand and kissed it, and she awoke. Conor's mother reached for Conor, and he took her hand. The yew tree monster, behind Conor, said, "*If you speak the truth . . . you will be able to face whatever comes.*"[47] Conor knew that the yew tree monster had come for this exact moment. And Conor spoke his personal truth:

> "I don't want you to go," he said, the tears dropping from his eyes, slowly at first, then spilling like a river.
> "I know, my love," his mother said in her heavy voice. "I know."
> He could feel the [yew tree] monster, holding him up and letting him stand there.
> "I don't want you to go," he said again.[48]

"And that," Ness writes, "was all that he needed to say."[49] Conor held his mother, tightly, and by "doing so, he could finally let her go."[50]

A Psychoanalytic Interpretation of a Dream in A Monster Calls

Each of the chapters in this book offers a theological bioethics that is psychologically-sophisticated, therapeutically-oriented, and experientially-grounded. This chapter is experientially-grounded by focusing on the case of Conor, thus building on the substantial tradition of literature and medicine. In terms of psychological and therapeutic inquiry, the focus of my analysis will be on one of the three stories that the yew tree monster tells (for a more detailed analysis that focuses on all three of the stories, see my longer article[51]) informed by Freud's theory of dreams.

In 1901 Freud published "On Dreams,"[52] a summary of the major insights from *The Interpretation of Dreams*.[53] By following the free associations of his patients and by examining his own dreams, Freud discovered that the meaning of a dream can be determined by following a certain interpretive method. For Freud the key to understanding dreams is that they should be understood as wishes. He gives this example:

> One day a girl of three and a quarter made a trip across a lake. The voyage was evidently not long enough for her, for she cried when she

> had to get off the boat. . . . [The next day] she reported that during the night she had been for a trip on the lake: she had been continuing her interrupted voyage [in her sleep during a dream].[54]

These kinds of dreams, which children often have (and adults sometimes do as well), can be seen as fulfilled wishes in the present. In this sense dreams help children and adults keep sleeping. If, for example, one is hungry before going to bed, one may dream about food so as not to wake from hunger. Dreams preserve sleep.

But not all dreams are understood as easily as this. Many dreams are strange. This is because the wish that is being expressed in the dream is disguised. Why? This disguising is due to the fact that the wish is unacceptable to the dreamer, often because the wish is sexual or aggressive in nature. This insight—that many dreams consist of wishes that are disguised—led Freud to postulate that dreams have two kinds of content: manifest content and latent content. The manifest content of a dream is the dream as we remember it when we wake up, but the latent content of the dream is the source of the dream. There is a mental process (what Freud called the dream-work) that converts the latent content of dreams into the manifest content of dreams.

The dream-work has a number of ways of converting the latent content of dreams into the manifest content of dreams. One is *condensation*. Here, various elements of a dream are compressed into a single construction. For condensation to work there "must be one or more *common elements* in all the components . . . [and] the common element in them then stands out clearly in the composite picture."[55] Freud adds:

> There are many sorts of ways in which figures . . . can be put together. I may build up a figure by giving it the features of two people; or I may give it the *form* of one person but think of it in the dream as having the *name* of another person; or I may have a visual picture of one person, but put it in a situation which is appropriate to another.[56]

Freud suggests that the dream-work often represents contrary ideas by the same composite structure and also that single elements of any given dream are "overdetermined"—that is, they do not have a single cause or meaning.

Another way that the dream-work has of converting the latent content of dreams into the manifest content of dreams is by means of *displacement*. Displacement in dreams occurs when "*psychical intensity passes over from the thoughts and ideas to which it properly belongs on to others which in our judgement have no claim to any such emphasis.*"[57] If a person were to dream of assassinating the king, for example, this may be an example of a wish to murder one's father. The mechanism of displacement also explains why dreams can be convoluted: "The more obscure and confused a dream appears to be, the greater the share in its construction that may be attributed to the factor of displacement."[58]

Dreams undergo various forms of distortion because such dreams are derived from repressed material, which is unconscious. When one is sleeping, one's critical agency[59] is weakened, thus allowing repressed material, in disguised form, to come to consciousness. This is why, in part, we forget our dreams shortly after we wake: Our critical agencies are fully functioning again. Freud also observes that there are three types of dreams: (i) dreams derived from unrepressed material that are not disguised and are easily understandable (e.g., as in the dream of the little girl previously mentioned who wanted to continue her voyage); (ii) dreams derived from repressed material that are disguised by means of the processes of the dream-work; and (iii) dreams derived from repressed material that is insufficiently disguised. This third type of dreams explains anxiety dreams. In such cases, the repressed wish is too close to becoming fully conscious so one wakes up instead of expressing the wish in the dream. Conor's waking up from the recurring nightmare illustrates this nicely.

While all of Conor's dreams (i.e., stories told by the yew tree monster) in *A Monster Calls* could be interpreted in light of Freud's theory, an interpretation of one of them is sufficient to demonstrate the hermeneutical richness that psychoanalysis—which is a traditional tool of pastoral theology—can bring to bioethics. I will offer a psychoanalytic interpretation of the first story told by the yew tree monster. This dream occurred after Conor's grandmother had come to visit to help take care of Conor's mother while she received another round of chemotherapy. What follows is a brief summary of the story told by the yew tree monster with my interpretation.

Once upon a time there was a town with a king who was wise on account of his suffering. The king's wife had given birth to four sons, but all of them died during various battles fought on behalf of the kingdom. One heir remained, the king's infant grandson. Then the king's wife died, as did the mother of the king's grandson (i.e., the king's daughter-in-law). So the king decided to remarry. He married a young princess from a neighboring kingdom.

As time passed, the royal infant grew into a young man, and the king grew ill. Some suspected that the king's new wife was poisoning him, and rumor had it that she was not young at all, that she was a witch who used magic to make herself appear to be young. The king died. The king's new wife became the queen, assuming the throne before the king's grandson, serving as regent in his place until he turned eighteen. She seemed to be a good queen.

Meanwhile, the prince fell in love. While most approved of this match, the queen did not, as she wanted to marry the prince so as to remain in power. But the prince refused to marry the queen (i.e., his stepmother), and he ran away with his beloved, vowing to return on his eighteenth birthday to free the kingdom from the queen.

One night the prince and his beloved slept together under a yew tree, and when the prince awoke, his love was dead. The prince ran back toward the village and told the townsfolk that the queen had killed his beloved. Enraged, the villagers stormed the queen's castle, and the yew tree monster marched with them. As the villagers were about to burn the queen alive, the yew tree monster picked the queen up and took her to safety, to a village far away by the sea, where she lived happily ever after.

Conor was furious. He wanted the queen to be punished for killing the prince's bride-to-be. But the yew tree monster told Conor that the queen did *not* kill her, even though the prince *said* that the queen did. The yew tree monster then told Conor that the prince killed his bride-to-be. Conor was baffled. The yew tree monster added that the prince himself told him that he had done so for the good of the kingdom, because the prince knew that he needed the help of the villagers to overthrow the queen. The prince reasoned that the only way to overthrow the queen was to murder his bride-to-be, framing the queen, so as to stir the anger of the villagers.

The yew tree monster said that the queen was indeed a witch but that she was not a murderer. Conor asked what happened to the prince (who became the king), if he ever got caught. The king lived happily ever after, too, the yew tree monster said. Conor, further upset and more confused, wondered what the lesson of this story was supposed to be. The yew tree monster said that in life most people are a mix of both good and bad. Conor greatly disliked the story. But the yew tree monster said it was nevertheless *true*.

Conor, identifying the witch in his story with his grandmother, asked the yew tree monster how he was going to save him from her. The yew tree monster replied that it is not his grandmother from whom he needs saving. Conor awoke from the dream.

The Oedipal resonances in this story are readily apparent. A (step)mother wishing to marry a (step)son is a reversal of the universal wish of a son wanting to marry his mother, taking the place of his father, using violence if necessary to do so. Symbols—for example, a king or a queen—are being used as disguising mechanisms of the dream-work. Also according to the dynamics of the dream-work, the murderous desire of the son in this story is displaced: The prince kills his bride-to-be, neither the father (who is already dead) nor his (step)mother. The fact that the queen can be seen as standing for various persons in Conor's psychic life—his father, his grandmother—suggests that condensation is at work here as well.

Also, the queen seems to stand for Conor's grandmother: Just as the queen wishes to marry the prince, so does Conor's grandmother want Conor to move in with her. The yew tree monster in the dream does indeed save Conor (the prince) from this fate, though not by killing the queen (his conscious wish to be free from his grandmother), but by saving her, removing her from the situation. The prince also gets away with killing his bride-to-be. This is unacceptable to Conor's conscious mind, but, to his unconscious mind, this is very healing. Why? This is because the prince's bride-to-be seems to stand for Conor's mother: Conor wishes to kill her and not be punished, just like the prince. He wants to be forgiven for wanting his mother to die.

As with most dreams, various principles of dream interpretation are at work, and there is not just one wish that is being expressed—that is, the dream is overdetermined. In sum, here are some of the apparent wishes:

1. the wish to have one's mother sexually (symbolized by means of the prince sleeping with his bride-to-be);
2. the wish to kill one's father to have one's mother (symbolized by means of the prince's plot to kill the queen); and
3. Conor's wish to kill his mother (symbolized by means of the prince murdering his bride-to-be).

Some of the wishes are contradictory, but this is not a problem for the dream-work. Indeed, the dream-work is attempting to express ambivalence—opposites—so contradiction is the rule, not the exception, in dream interpretation. For Conor, who is suffering from profound ambivalence (i.e., he is holding mutually exclusive wishes, with no rational way of resolving them), the dream frees him from this ambivalence by expressing it in disguised form, in the form of paradox: the wicked queen is saved, not punished, by the yew tree monster.

What Does This Psychoanalytic Interpretation Add?

My point in offering this inquiry into Conor's dream is to explore, with specific theoretical tools commonly used by pastoral theologians, Boisen's claim that "the mind [can become] dominated by [an] idea which [it] has been trying to put in its proper place."[60] For Conor, this idea was the impending death of his mother, something he both feared and wanted. Freud's insights regarding dreams give us a particular way of exploring persons as living human documents. Of note, without a great deal of attention given to Conor's life, a psychoanalytic interpretation would not be compelling. Indeed, this amount of space puts me in a position to offer some implications of the correlation of respect for autonomy and the living human document for bioethics in light of psychoanalysis.

A Pastoral Perspective on Respect for Autonomy

For Beauchamp and Childress, respect for autonomy is about choice. Applying this principle in clinical, research, and public health settings often entails thinking through situations where it may not be obvious who should decide, as the Quinlan case illustrated. As a centric force in bioethics, principlist applications of respect for autonomy tend to focus on, as previously detailed, issues such as informed consent, truth-telling, privacy and confidentially, and capacity and competency issues.

In each chapter providing a correlation, I will offer one way of looking at a principle through the lens of pastoral theology (via an image of pastoral care), and I will describe what difference this correlation makes, concluding with a practical illustration of what I envision as an operationalization of this correlation. My suggestion in this chapter is this: *A pastoral perspective on respect for autonomy shifts the focus away from a respect of choice to an appreciation of individuals.* In a sense, this suggestion recovers the roots of this principle in the Belmont Report when it was named respect for persons (not respect for autonomy).[61] While principlist bioethics has been criticized for focusing too much on respect for autonomy, some of this criticism can be softened by recovering this older way of understanding the principle.

Respecting persons as individuals has a long tradition in pastoral theology. Indeed, this is what the living human document is all about. In *Giving Counsel: A Minister's Guidebook*, Donald Capps suggests that in providing one with counsel the most important thing is having "a judicious frame of mind."[62] For Capps this entails, in part, a particular way of being kind. Quoting

Kelly Cannon's *Henry James and Masculinity: The Man at the Margins*, Capps writes: "To be genuinely kind necessitates an appreciation of the complex life within every person,"[63] and he adds, even if this cannot be known, such an appreciation "is a precondition of being 'genuinely kind.'"[64]

In this chapter I have offered a psychoanalytic reading of *A Monster Calls* as a way of appreciating the complex life that exists within one person: Conor. I explored Conor's complex life by analyzing one of his dreams, a dream that expressed his profound ambivalence. *A Monster Calls*, precisely because it is a work of fiction, gives the reader a rich look into the dynamics of ambivalence, for as readers we know things about Conor that he does not know about himself.

While this focus on *A Monster Calls* provides a means of offering a thick account of moral experience, what does this have to do with respect for autonomy? On the surface, *A Monster Calls* seems to have little, if anything, to do with respect for autonomy because *A Monster Calls* is not about Conor's mother's clinical choices.

A different, and perhaps a straightforward, choice in this regard would have been a piece of fiction such as *Wit*,[65] a play that later became a film. *Wit* is about a professor going through an experimental trial to treat cancer, and *Wit* has been very influential in bioethics teaching because it raises many of the centric issues of bioethics previously noted in a contextualized (i.e., thick) manner. In contrast to *A Monster Calls, Wit* deals directly with the protagonist's choices and issues of informed consent.[66]

But I have chosen *A Monster Calls* precisely because this enables me to offer a fresh perspective. Indeed, correlating the principles with atypical literature choices opens up new possibilities for creativity where literature is not merely an instrument for illustration but is instead a source of imagination.[67] Focusing on Conor—instead of a work such as *Wit*—demonstrates the shift from respecting choices (the traditional focus of principlist bioethics regarding respect for autonomy) to appreciating individuals (this pastoral perspective on respect for autonomy) because for Conor there is no medical decision to be made, no informed consent document to be signed. What psychoanalysis adds is a method of appreciating individuality. Also, illness strikes not only patients but also families; this particular correlation highlights this fact.

So, again, if respecting the autonomy of persons in light of the living human document means appreciating persons as individuals, taking insights from psychoanalysis is one way of doing so. There are other ways. What psychoanalysis adds specifically to this discussion is that patients who are competent and who do have capacity are nevertheless not always rational because they are motivated by unconscious forces. This is important because principlist bioethics tends to assume people are rational actors, and, if not, they do not have capacity. Yet I am not suggesting that health professionals ought to psychoanalyze their patients or the family members of their patients. What I am making a case for, rather, is more modest: I think that caregivers should assume complexity in the lives of their patients (and their families) and that caregivers should be curious about this complexity.

To put this another way, the key take away for health professionals regarding my psychoanalytic reading of *A Monster Calls* is for them to assume that patients and their family members often experience ambivalence about their choices. Perhaps this is especially so when the stakes are high, when the decisions are life and death. We all need to be patient with patients as well as with their family members, assuming not rational actors who can make autonomous choices but assuming instead ambivalent individuals who do not know what they want, because they want opposite things at the same time.

A Final Illustration: The African Violet Queen

Because *A Monster Calls* is fiction, the reader has every right to ask: What might appreciating persons as individuals look like in actual practice? I address this question by concluding with a case from Milton Erickson, a well-known American psychiatrist who was interested in unconscious processes and also an advocate of brief therapy. While he was controversial—one of his more controversial cases will be discussed in chapter 4—this case, referred to by Capps as "The African Violet Queen," is not so much controversial as it is uplifting.

One of Erickson's students asked him to help a woman who had made several suicide attempts:

> Instead of attempting to arrange an appointment at his office, Erickson simply showed up at the woman's home . . . where she lived alone with her maid. When she came to the door, he introduced himself and asked to be given a tour of the house. Surprised but intrigued, she agreed to show him around.
>
> In the sun porch, he noticed a row of pots containing African violets. The lady informed him that the one thing she had a touch for was growing these plants. He also learned that she went to church every Sunday, but other than that had no meaningful social life. Upon

> leaving . . . he said to her, "Madame, here is your prescription. I want you to send your maid to the nursery to purchase many more pots and every strain of African violets they carry. Furthermore, whenever a child is born to a member of your congregation, I want you to give a pot of African violets to the parents at the baptism. And whenever a wedding is celebrated, I want you to give a pot of these flowers to the bride."[68]

Capps notes that the woman went on to live for another twenty years, dying at the age of seventy-six. He adds that this vignette illustrates Erickson's practice of entering the patient's world by using the patient's own language. Specifically, Erickson noticed in this woman two things that gave her meaning in life—gardening and religion—and he linked the two for her in a creative way. Capps writes: "By connecting them, he addressed her suicidal threats, which derived from her feeling that her life lacked any real purpose. By entering her world he was able to work within her own frame of life and not impose his onto hers."[69] When the woman died, the local newspaper titled her obituary: "The African Violet Queen Dies at Age 76." It told of her dedication to church and kindness to others.

If principlist bioethics as a centric force likely would focus on this woman's lack of capacity with regard to her suicidal ideation (the clinical issue in the foreground of the patient's life), perhaps leading to an involuntary hospitalization, a pastoral perspective on respect for autonomy, as an eccentric force, would focus on what usually are thought of as marginal details of a patient's history: church attendance and gardening (features in the background of the patient's life). Indeed, while Erickson could have sought involuntary hospitalization, thus temporarily suspending this woman's autonomy, he instead studied her as a living human document—and saved her life.

Like Conor, this woman experienced some kind of "disorganization," to use Boisen's term, of her world. She, like Conor, was falling apart, and Erickson helped this woman find meaning, as did the yew tree monster for Conor. While both my interpretation of Conor and Erickson's interpretation of this woman recognized unconscious motivations, what was healing for this woman was not prolonged therapy but rather an act of kindness: a prescription of meaning. Erickson's kindness was specific to her; he appreciated her as an individual.

While I think the primary motivation for viewing patients as living human documents is to provide better care, I hope this call to curiosity also will stimulate the moral imaginations of caregivers, enabling them to reconnect to why their work is so deeply meaningful, if reconnection is needed. If caregivers find themselves losing empathy for patients and if they find themselves experiencing burnout due to a variety of reasons (especially time constraints and financial pressures), ultimately becoming disconnected from why they pursued this life as a health professional in the first place, I wonder if viewing patients as living human documents, as having experiential depth, would make a difference? Would this enable encounters to become an opportunity to witness the complexity of what it means to be an individual? Would this yield some healing for healers, who also are living human documents in need of care? I hope so.

3 NONMALEFICENCE AND THE CIRCUS CLOWN

Atul Gawande, a surgeon and best-selling author who writes regularly for the *New Yorker* and other such venues, begins *Complications: A Surgeon's Notes on an Imperfect Science*, a finalist for a national book award, by writing about an occasion on trauma duty when a young man, about twenty years old, presented with a gunshot wound.[1] All of his vital signs were fine. While the entrance wound was readily apparent, Gawande observed, there did not appear to be an exit wound, meaning that the bullet was still inside of him. Also, when Gawande did the rectal exam, he found blood. He did again when he inserted a urinary catheter into him. All of this suggested internal bleeding; the patient would die without immediate surgery. When Gawande explained this to the patient, he reluctantly agreed, despite the fact that he felt fine. Surgery was necessary to save this young man's life.

Or so Gawande thought. "We made a fast, deep slash down the middle of his abdomen, from his rib cage to his pubis," Gawande writes, and "we grabbed the retractors and pulled him open. And what we found was . . . nothing."[2] Amazingly, there was no internal bleeding. And when they checked the catheter again, there was no blood there either. They also could not find the bullet, despite searching for an hour. Moreover, there was no trace of the bullet on the X-rays. They sewed him back up.

A couple of days later, however, Gawande's team received another X-ray, and this one *did* show that the bullet was still inside him. Gawande reflects, "We had no explanation for any of this—how a half-inch-long lead bullet had gotten from his buttock to his upper belly without injuring anything, why it hadn't appeared on the previous X-rays, or where the blood we had seen had come from. Having already done more harm than the bullet had, however, we left it and the young man alone. We kept him in the hospital for a week. Except for our gash, he turned out fine."[3]

This clinical vignette provides a clear introduction to the principle of nonmaleficence. It highlights the fact that medicine is a human—and therefore a messy, uncertain, and fallible—endeavor, just as much as it is a science (though science also, to be sure, is messy, uncertain, and fallible). In this case, the patient was harmed by the surgery that was inflicted upon him, and it seems as though he would have been better off had he been left alone. Still, Gawande and his team did the right thing because it was very likely that the young man was bleeding internally from the gunshot wound. It is hard to imagine any surgeon making a different choice than the one that Gawande did. But the decision to do nothing further (other than a week of observation) was grounded in nonmaleficence.

Part One: The Principle

The focus of this chapter is on nonmaleficence. In part one I begin by providing an overview of the principle and then review a classic case in bioethics on abortion to illustrate how the principle is often understood. I also draw on poetry to intimate that moral issues beyond decision-making are relevant to abortion. Then in part two I offer a discussion of Heije Faber's pastoral image of the circus clown to set the stage for opening up another way of looking at nonmaleficence. The essential feature of Faber's image for my purposes is that it provides a theological rationale for appreciating humor in the hospital. In part three, I correlate nonmaleficence and the circus clown by using an essay by Sigmund Freud on humor to interpret select passages from scenes from two pathographies. My argument is that a pastoral perspective on nonmaleficence can help to mitigate harm stemming from idolatry.

Nonmaleficence

Beauchamp and Childress state plainly that "the principle of nonmaleficence obligates us to abstain from causing harm to others."[4] They add that a celebrated maxim in medical ethics is "First, do no harm," a maxim falsely attributed to the Hippocratic corpus.[5] In exploring this principle key topics include:

- killing and allowing to die,
- intending and foreseeing harmful outcomes,
- withholding and withdrawing life-sustaining treatments,
- extraordinary and ordinary treatments,

- the underproduction as well as the overprotection of human subjects, and
- advance directives and surrogate decision-making.

They also add that nonmaleficence entails intentional avoidance of actions that cause harm.

Beauchamp and Childress note a distinction between harming and wronging, in that one can be harmed without being wronged, and vice versa. For example, one can be physically harmed from a hurricane but not morally wronged. Or a patient can be wronged by an insurance company if the insurance company denies a legitimate claim for which the hospital assumes the cost—this is being wronged without being harmed. Beauchamp and Childress define harm as "a thwarting, defeating, or setting back of some party's interests," but they add that "a harmful action is not always a wrong or unjustified."[6] An example they offer in this regard is the amputation of a patient's leg to save his or her life. What nonmaleficence requires is not the complete avoidance of harm but rather a justification of harmful actions inflicted. Nonmaleficence also includes the obligation not to impose risks of harm, including negligence. If a nurse were to not change a bandage at a scheduled time (and therefore increase the risk of infection) nonmaleficence would be violated.

Regarding the distinction between withholding and withdrawing treatments, withholding refers to not starting a given treatment and withdrawing refers to stopping treatments that have already started. A common belief among health professionals and family members alike is that it is morally permissible to withhold treatment, but withdrawing treatment (such as disconnecting a ventilator) is another matter. Philosophers tend to discount the ambiguities of the distinction between withdrawing and withholding treatment: "Feelings of reluctance about withdrawing treatments are understandable," Beauchamp and Childress write, "but the distinction between withdrawing and withholding treatments is morally irrelevant and potentially dangerous."[7] However, in clinical practice it is sometimes ambiguous as to whether restarting a treatment—such as reinserting a central line that has become dislodged—is withholding or withdrawing. Relatedly, the difficulty of the procedure might influence one's assessment in this regard.

A problem with prioritizing withholding treatment over withdrawing treatment, Beauchamp and Childress argue, is that this can lead to both overtreatment (because it is difficult to stop treatment once it has begun) *and* undertreatment (because families do not want to be trapped in a medical system that tilts toward the continuation of treatment once it has begun).

Also, Beauchamp and Childress reject the distinction between ordinary and extraordinary treatment because, they claim, it is "unacceptably vague and morally misleading."[8] They argue that a key distinction that should matter—as opposed to usual/unusual, simple/complex, natural/artificial, noninvasive/highly invasive, inexpensive/expensive, routine/heroic, and so on—is beneficial or burdensome.

Another common distinction, which is key for the doctrine of double effect, involves intended effects and foreseen effects. The doctrine of double effect states that a single action—such as the administering of a large dose of morphine—may have both a beneficial effect and a harmful effect and that this action is not morally wrong as long as the harmful effect was not intended even though it was foreseen. Thus, a doctor may not give a large dose of morphine with the intention of killing a patient. However, a doctor may give a patient a large dose of morphine with the intention of relieving pain, while also foreseeing likely death. Beauchamp and Childress reject distinctions that rely on intention because they are unobservable and unknowable.

Another distinction that Beauchamp and Childress favor is between optional treatments and obligatory treatments. While there is a prima facie obligation to treat patients appearing to need medical attention, this obligation can be overridden when the treatment is determined to be futile[9] or when the burdens of treatment outweigh the benefits (i.e., quality-of-life considerations). Relatedly, Beauchamp and Childress discuss the distinction between killing and letting die. They argue that one cannot assess the rightness or wrongness of either without context, unlike in cases of murder, which is always wrong. The language that Beauchamp and Childress prefer is not killing or letting die but rather intentionally arranging death.[10]

While most of the chapter focuses on clinical ethics, Beauchamp and Childress also discuss a research ethics case involving Native Americans. The research was conducted by Arizona State University. Since the 1960s, a particular tribe experienced a high incidence of type 2 diabetes, which led to a high rate of amputations within the tribe. Leaders from the tribe were very interested when approached by researchers in the 1990s, hoping that by providing deoxyribonucleic acid (DNA) samples something could be learned about their tribe's genetics to help them. The consent form for the study stated that the research was to study "the causes of behavioral/medical disorders."[11]

The study enrolled about one hundred research participants. Diabetes was studied, but schizophrenia and the effects of inbreeding within the tribe were studied as well. Nearly two dozen articles were published resulting from this research. When the tribe found out about these publications, they filed a lawsuit, claiming that they only consented to diabetes research. They felt that the other research was "offensive, insulting, stigmatizing, harmful, and provocative."[12] The university subsequently issued payment to the tribe for "wrong that was done."[13] Beauchamp and Childress argue that the case points to a need for a "richer conception of harms in research than often occurs. Research on samples, especially genetics research, can create psychosocial risks in the absence of physical risks to individual sources of the samples."[14]

They close the chapter with a discussion of how to protect patients who lack capacity. This falls under the rubric of nonmaleficence because "protecting patients from negligence and harm is the central issue."[15] Advance directives, in the form of living wills as well as designations for a proxy to hold durable power of attorney, are discussed. Much of the space that they give to exploring this principle deals with issues related to end-of-life care, with an emphasis on mitigating harm resulting from medical treatment and research studies.

An Illustration: The Case of Alice Roe

The case that I use in this chapter to illustrate nonmaleficence involves abortion. While, as noted, the Hippocratic Oath does not contain the phrase "do no harm," various versions of the oath do contain a prohibition against abortion,[16] so the association of this principle with abortion has historical precedent.

Abortion has been a hotly debated topic in bioethics for decades. In a sense, one might understand the debate as centered on which harm should count for more: the human fetus's or the woman's? Peter Singer has observed that opinions on both sides have not been altered very much, and he has outlined the formal argument against abortion as follows:

> First premise: It is wrong to kill an innocent human being.
> Second premise: A human fetus is an innocent human being.
> Conclusion: Therefore, it is wrong to kill a human fetus.[17]

Singer notes that most of the debate over abortion concerns the second premise, about whether the fetus is a human being (or "life"). He thinks that this premise is difficult to refute, as the fetus is obviously alive, and, if it is not human, then what is it? The conclusion that the fetus is a human life seems inescapable and unshakable. It would seem to be difficult to refute the innocence of the fetus as well.

Singer's contribution to this debate is that he disputes the first premise, that it is wrong to kill an innocent human being. As a utilitarian, Singer does not think that any act, in and of itself, is inherently wrong because actions should be judged by their consequences. In cases where killing an innocent human being would bring about more happiness on the whole and in the long run, such killing would be justified. For Singer this includes not only killing fetuses (abortion) but also killing babies (infanticide). That Singer permits the killing of babies in some limited circumstances is one of his more controversial positions.[18]

In this chapter I would like to discuss the issue of abortion more concretely and to do so I turn to a classic case. The case involves Kenneth Edelin, the first physician to be brought up on legal charges in the United States for performing an abortion after *Roe v. Wade*, a landmark legal case that permits some forms of abortion.

In 1973 Edelin was a third-year resident at Boston City Hospital, and he was involved with the case of Alice Roe (not her real name). Very little is known about Alice. At the time, Alice was seventeen, and she presented with a request for an abortion. There was some disagreement as to whether she was twenty-two or twenty-four weeks pregnant because the hospital did not have an ultrasound machine. Hugh Holtrop, who was Edelin's faculty supervisor, assigned the abortion to Edelin. Gregory Pence writes:

> Edelin planned to abort Alice Roe's fetus by injecting saline solution into the amniotic sac, but when he inserted a needle . . . to sample the amniotic fluid, he drew blood. This indicated that the patient had an anterior placenta (that is, a placenta attached to the front wall of the uterus); thus a saline solution injected into the placenta could travel from there into her bloodstream, where it could be lethal [to the mother].[19]

The abortion was rescheduled for the following day so that a hysterectomy could be performed. Pence notes that the following account of this procedure is controversial. A resident who witnessed the procedure testified that "Edelin made the cesarean section, reached in, cut the placenta from the abdominal wall, then waited perhaps 3 minutes, and after this interval removed a dead fetus."[20] Pence adds, "If such a wait took place, that would be important, because a baby cannot breathe on its own inside the uterus: It begins breathing (if at all) only when it is brought out. Edelin would later be charged with 'neglecting' the baby by not removing it immediately, thus causing it to suffocate."[21] For this reason Edelin was charged with manslaughter. (I would like to add here that, while Singer's views on infanticide may have seemed extreme and unrealistic, this clinical case illustrates that the line between abortion and infanticide can be thin.)

Pence notes that the trial judge described the charge as follows: "The essence of wanton or reckless conduct is the doing of an act or the omission to act where there is a duty to act, which commission or omission involves a high degree of likelihood that substantial harm will result to another."[22] Thus, one can see that the moral principle of nonmaleficence and the legal definition of manslaughter are closely related. Edelin was found guilty and charged with a year of probation. He also could have lost his medical license, but the conviction was overturned by a higher court about three years later and he was acquitted.

While the moral and legal status of abortion in the United States and perhaps elsewhere remains opaque, questions relating to nonmaleficence are clearer: Who is being harmed? What is the harm? Whose harm counts for more? How serious is the harm? How is this seriousness assessed? Is there more than one harm? Are these harms being performed for a greater good? How is this greater good being calculated? Whom will these harms benefit? These questions are not only relevant to abortion in particular but also to applications of nonmaleficence in general.

Richer Conceptions of Harm

I previously noted that Beauchamp and Childress argue that there is a need for richer conceptions of harm. While they were writing specifically about research ethics, their observation can apply across the board. With regard to abortion, such a richer conception of harm can be explored by turning to medical humanist Marilyn McEntyre and her use of poetry.

In *Patient Poets* McEntyre observes, "Though it gets so much press as a legal and moral issue, the actual experience of abortion, its physical process and psychological costs, are still less freely discussed than the abstractions in which we more readily clothe it when we discuss it as a theological controversy or legal problem."[23] She continues:

> Even among those who, as a matter of political conviction, support women's right to choose abortion, conversation about personal experiences of abortion can be riddled with emotional pain, ambivalence, guilt, and grief. The loss of something more consequential than

> blood and tissue is undeniable for the woman who has just traveled the steep trajectory of feeling from lovemaking to pregnancy test to decision-making to clinic.[24]

McEntyre offers Anne Sexton's poem "The Abortion" to give voice to various types of emotion related to abortion. (I strongly encourage the reader to pause, google the poem, and read it now; it is available online in many places.) She discusses a number of aspects of the poem but what I want to highlight here are her comments about the ending of the poem: "The issue upon which the poem concludes is not the morality of abortion—whether or not it is murder—but the matter of moral courage that is required even of those who have made the decision and carried it through."[25] She adds:

> To admit that what has happened is a real death, that what is lost is a real life, is not necessarily to conclude that it should not have been done, but certainly that to do it exacts an ethical struggle and a psychological cost. The temptation to minimize, explain away, or pretend, and the consequences of doing any of those, the poem suggests, are [at] least as significant a matter for the one who makes the decision as are theoretical arguments about the rightness or wrongness of the decision itself.[26]

Thus, what McEntyre has offered here is a richer account of the premise that Singer freely passes over, namely, that a human fetus is an innocent human being. McEntyre's discussion of Sexton's poem demonstrates the plurality and the complexity of the moral concerns regarding abortion. Indeed, there are *many* moral concerns regarding abortion, many harms worth our inquiry, especially harms that cannot be explored abstractly but rather only personally and in context.[27] Continuing from the main theological claim from chapter 2 and also inspired by an influential feminist slogan, the personal is theological.[28] Sexton's poem invites the reader to ask: How do we care for women who have had abortions—psychologically, emotionally, and socially? How do we care for them religiously, spiritually, and ecclesiologically?[29]

Part Two: The Image

Having provided an overview of nonmaleficence as well as an illustration of it, I now want to turn to the circus clown to set the stage for offering a pastoral perspective on nonmaleficence.

The Circus Clown

In "The Circus Clown," Faber writes about hospital chaplaincy.[30] As such, this image is especially appropriate for bioethics. Faber compares ministers with clowns, but in doing so he by no means wishes to degrade ministers or chaplains, for clowns are a necessity in the circus—without whom the circus would not be a circus.

Faber suggests that the main appeal of clowns is that they give us perspective, for the circus is a

> place in which people perform great feats, tame wild animals, and do hair-raising stunts on the trapeze. They [i.e., these acts] make us feel tense and frightened, but the clown puts it back in perspective. In a childish way he makes these stuntmen look a little foolish; he makes us feel that they are, after all, only human and ordinary, and thus re-establishes a sort of spiritual balance.[31]

He goes on to note that, while the clown is a part of the team, he or she is essentially alone, having "a kind of solidarity with the public in the boundary situations of our existence: sorrow, the absurd, setbacks."[32]

The chaplain, likewise, is a part of the team and like the clown does not have impressive skills when compared with the nurse or the surgeon. Faber writes:

> The hospital is the scene of tremendous feats; between these walls great strides are made in the march of science and technology. Those working there are all experts in their own fields who have had a special training for their task. The specialists, nurses, social workers, analysts, physiotherapists—they are all trapeze-artistes, but the poor clergyman is the clown. He presents a clear contrast to all of them.[33]

"The minister," he adds "is only true to his[34] calling when he does not draw attention to himself in any way whatever but, by his actions and his words, points a way to the one in whose service he stands, whom he represents and seeks to make present to the man in his sickness."[35] In other words, chaplains should not attempt to become like other health professionals who *do* things. Why? For chaplains, their *being* is their calling. "What matters," Faber writes, "is his attitude, whether he has a real interest in . . . the patients, the staff, in all concerned, in the institution itself."[36]

In the hospital, the chaplain (from a Christian perspective) is a representative of the church and of Christ, and Faber relays a remark from a surgeon about what chaplains add.

> We need the minister for the climate, the spirit of the hospital. It is not that we want to have a certain reputation, that with us, as in church hospitals, there are services and that we therefore meet the wishes of those patients who value them; it is, rather, that we recognize that our medical work comes to stand in a different framework when the minister works beside us, a framework which we sense to be right.[37]

Part Three: Correlation of Principle and Image

As noted, each of the chapters in this book offers inquiry that is theologically-informed, psychologically-sophisticated, therapeutically-oriented, and experientially-grounded, and this is accomplished by correlating a bioethics principle and a pastoral image. To explore the possibilities of correlating nonmaleficence with the circus clown, I turn to two cases: the case of Jean-Dominique Bauby (from a best-selling memoir about locked-in syndrome[38]) and the case of Jason Micheli (from a recent book about a pastor's struggle with a rare form of cancer[39]). This provides experiential material. In the previous chapter I employed fiction as a means of moral inquiry. Here, I turn to memoir. In the memoirs I focus on scenes that deal with humor, and I interpret these scenes by using an essay on humor by Freud as a means to incorporate psychological and therapeutic perspectives into the correlation, just as in chapter 2.

In terms of the structure of this correlation, I begin with Bauby's experience to introduce issues of humor in clinical settings, turn to Freud for initial hermeneutical insights regarding humor, and then return to experience again—Micheli's experience—to explore more fully the place of humor in clinical encounters. After this psychological, therapeutic, and experiential inquiry, I offer a pastoral perspective on nonmaleficence that is explicitly theological. Also, I would like to emphasize my belief that it is important to privilege the perspective of patients when discussing the role of humor in the hospital (especially when the patients are dealing with diseases as deadly as these) because the possibilities for humiliation are too great.

The Case of Jean-Dominique Bauby

In *The Diving Bell and the Butterfly*, Jean-Dominique Bauby, former editor of the prestigious French magazine *Elle*, describes his life after a stroke that left him suffering from locked-in syndrome when he was just forty-three. He died two days after the book was published, shortly before turning forty-five. The title of the book refers to how he experiences his life in locked-in syndrome: "My heels hurt, my head weighs a ton, and something like a giant invisible diving bell holds my whole body prisoner."[40] Sometimes, though, "my diving bell becomes less oppressive, and my mind takes flight like a butterfly. There is so much to do. You can wander off in space or in time."[41]

Bauby notes that locked-in syndrome is the result of medical progress: "In the past . . . you simply died. But improved resuscitation techniques have now prolonged and refined the agony. . . . Paralyzed from head to toe, the patient, his mind intact, is imprisoned inside his own body, unable to speak or move."[42] This is the key issue for nonmaleficence in many countries today: medical technology can inflict more harm than it relieves suffering. Bauby adds that in his case blinking his left eyelid was his only means of communication. Remarkably, he wrote the entire memoir by blinking to communicate letters to a transcriber.

Bauby underscores that it took time, as one might expect, for him to understand and to accept his diagnosis and prognosis. Previously he had grandiose plans, but eventually he had to give them up, with his new goal simply being able to swallow the saliva in his mouth. Not only was he forced to develop new goals and with these a new self-image, but also he was confronted with a new physical image of himself, one which was utterly foreign to him:

> Reflected in the glass I saw the head of a man who seemed to have emerged from a vat of formaldehyde. His mouth was twisted, his nose damaged, his hair tousled, his gaze full of fear. One eye was sewn shut, the other goggled like the doomed eye of Cain. For a moment I stared at the dilated pupil, before I realized it was only mine.[43]

He continues:

> Whereupon a strange euphoria came over me. Not only was I exiled, paralyzed, mute, half deaf, deprived of all pleasures, and reduced to

> the existence of a jellyfish, but I was also horrible to behold. There comes a time when the heaping up of calamities brings on uncontrollable nervous laughter—when, after a final blow from fate, we decide to treat it all as a joke.[44]

Bauby also writes about a certain "couldn't-care-less doctor" who is arrogant and rude. He ponders this doctor's perpetual clinical question to him: "Do you see double?"[45] He fantasizes about replying, "Yes, I see two assholes, not one."[46] Yet he feels that this asshole of a doctor provides him with a gift: the gift of enabling him to feel strongly. This is very important, he writes, because:

> I need to feel strongly, to love and to admire, just as desperately as I need to breathe. . . . [And] to keep my mind sharp, to avoid descending into resigned indifference, I maintain a level of resentment and anger, neither too much nor too little, just as a pressure cooker has a safety valve to keep it from exploding.[47]

The fact that he died just two days after the publication of his book could suggest that he lost the will to live. Writing the book sustained him, it seems, as did anger, and so too humor. But the fact that he died after completing the book suggests that humor, while valuable, nevertheless has limits. Humor is not meaning, and in extreme circumstances of suffering, meaning is required to endure.

The final chapter of the book, "Season of Renewal," recounts Bauby's observations about and experiences of the season of fall. He notes how much progress he has made both in speech therapy (he is now able to grunt a song) and with his book. The final scene of the book is with one of his caregivers, who helped him to write the book, and he observes that her purse is half open and in it he sees a subway ticket and a folded bill. Looking at these objects, he wonders if somewhere in the cosmos there is a ticket to buy his freedom—or if, instead, he is riding a subway that does not terminate. "We must keep looking," he writes, and the book ends.[48]

While the book has been generally praised, in *Signifying Bodies: Disability in Contemporary Life Writing*, G. Thomas Couser offers a strong critique of the book from a disabilities studies perspective.[49] Couser observes that the narrative arc of the book is one of recession, and therefore issues of accessibility are not addressed: "Although there is little that physicians can do for him other than to stabilize his condition and minimize his discomfort, his narrative in no way challenges the medical paradigm."[50] In other words, the memoir tends to reinforce ableism rather than challenge it.

A Psychoanalytic Inquiry into Humor

Freud had a long-standing interest in humor. Indeed, one of his earliest books was *Jokes and Their Relation to the Unconscious*,[51] published in 1905. In "Humor,"[52] published in 1928, Freud returns to the subject, revisiting it in light of some developments in his thinking about the mind. The key point in this essay is that he understands humor to be a function of the superego—a surprising and creative conclusion from Freud, given that Freud normally understands the superego to be a hard taskmaster.

Freud begins the essay by noting that in his previous work he analyzed humor from what he calls "an economic point of view."[53] By this he means that humor can save us from experiencing painful emotions such as fear and anxiety. Freud assumes that we all have limited psychic energy (just like we all have limited physical energy) and that humor is a more efficient way of spending psychic energy than other more costly ways. To demonstrate the economic effects of humor, Freud considers the listener of humor. The humorist tells the listener a story, which seems to be leading in the direction of anger, pain, or despair. The listener is prepared to feel these feelings with the storyteller. But just at the end of the story or joke, the humorist, instead of expressing painful emotions, jests. Freud writes: "The expenditure on feeling that is economized turns into humorous pleasure in the listener."[54]

Freud notes that there are two ways that humor can be expressed. One is when a person adopts a humorous attitude. Freud offers this joke as an example: "A criminal who was being led out to the gallows on a Monday remarked: 'Well, the week is beginning nicely.' "[55] As an observer to this remark, the onlooker also may derive pleasure from this joke. The other form of humor is between two people, when one person is the butt of a joke, such as a sarcastic remark (e.g., if someone misses a layup in basketball and an onlooker yells, "Nice shot!"). It is worth noting that there is a literature on the philosophy of humor.[56] This literature is beyond the scope of this chapter.

Freud goes on to note that humor has something liberating about it, which he attributes to a "triumph of narcissism," and he describes this as "the victorious assertion of the ego's invulnerability."[57] He adds: "It insists that it cannot be affected by the traumas of the external world; it shows, in fact, that such traumas are no more than occasions for it to gain pleasure."[58] Humor,

Freud continues, is not resigned but is rebellious. He returns, insightfully, to the previously offered joke to illustrate this:

> Let us suppose that the criminal who was being led to execution on Monday had said: "It doesn't worry me. What does it matter, after all, if a fellow like me is hanged? The world won't come to an end because of it." We should have to admit that such a speech does in fact display the same magnificent superiority over the real situation. It is wise and true; but it does not betray a trace of humor.[59]

Freud adds that humor seems to be close to other defense mechanisms that attempt to protect the ego But the difference is that humor does not begin with neurosis and lead to madness, as can happen when, for example, repression as a defense mechanism is employed.

Freud then goes on to understand humor in light of the superego. He notes that the superego is the nucleus of the ego and that the superego is "the heir to the parental agency."[60] Psychodynamically speaking, the mind consists of three components: the id, the ego, and the superego. At birth the mind consists only of the id, which is instinctual, and it is the part of us that seeks pleasure. In time the ego and the superego develop. The superego is derived from those who raise us (normally our parents). These persons put our id in check, telling us "no," "bad," "wait," "wrong," and so on. Thus, the superego forms our conscience. While a psychological concept (and therefore not observable via brain scans or dissections of the brain), the superego can be observed when persons exhibit guilt, shame, and regret. Freud typically thinks of the superego as the id's harsh critic. The ego provides the mind's executive function and attempts to mediate between the id and the superego. So, if the id pursues pleasure at all costs and if the superego demands perfection in all areas of life, the ego attempts to find more reasonable and realistic ways to live.

While one might have expected Freud to suggest that the ego employs humor as a defense mechanism to find a middle way between the id and the superego (Freud suggests that the ego employs a number of other defense mechanisms, such as denial, displacement, and projection), he asserted that the humorous attitude derives from the superego:

> We obtain a [psycho]dynamic [as opposed to economic] explanation of the humorous attitude, therefore, if we assume that it consists in the humorist's having withdrawn the psychical accent from his ego and

> having transposed it on to his superego. To the superego, thus inflated, the ego can appear tiny and all its interests trivial; and, with this new distribution of energy, it may become an easy matter for the superego to suppress the ego's possibility of reacting.[61]

It is as though the superego says to the ego: "'Look! Here is the world, which seems so dangerous! It is nothing but a game for children—just worth making a jest about!'"[62] Freud concludes this essay by noting:

> If it is really the superego which, in humor, speaks such kindly words of comfort to the intimated ego, this will teach us that we have still a great deal to learn about the nature of the superego. . . . And . . . if the superego tries, by means of humor, to console the ego and protect it from suffering, this does not contradict its origin in the parental agency.[63]

What Freud offers in this essay, then, is not only an explanation of *what* humor does (it saves us psychic energy) but also *how* this occurs (the superego acts like a kind parent to the overwhelmed ego).

Humor in The Diving Bell and the Butterfly

There is not much humor in *The Diving Bell and the Butterfly*. This is not surprising, for locked-in syndrome is no laughing matter. The humor in the book—the instance of horror turning into laughter as well as the instance when he referred to his doctor as an asshole—pretty much covers it. The former instance of humor can be understood as a defense mechanism. This man's image, a man whose life was dedicated to fashion, became in his own words "horrible to behold," and his response of laughter was not unlike the man headed for the gallows in Freud's joke. The man was about to die, and Bauby was indeed disfigured, but both of these occasions were for these men something to laugh about. Because life truly was too difficult for both men, their superego came to their ego's defense, telling them, in effect, that these matters are child's play.

The latter instance is a little different because it involves anger. Bauby notes insightfully that he needs to feel strongly to live, and feeling anger toward his doctor is one way of doing so. Feeling nothing but rage, however, would be exhausting—and too costly to the psyche from an economic point of view. The mixing of anger and humor here enables Bauby to feel strongly in an efficient way. This form of humor may be understood as a function of the superego as well, in that the superego is reacting against the misbehavior of another. It is as though the superego, as a protective parent to Bauby, is expressing disapproval of the mistreatment of his child (Bauby's ego) by the doctor, and this disapproval is expressed via sarcasm.

When a Harry Potter Dementor Sucks Your Soul Out of Your Ass

In *Cancer Is Funny: Keeping Faith in Stage-Serious Chemo*, Jason Micheli, a young pastor, husband, and father who was diagnosed with a rare and usually deadly form of cancer (mantle cell), offers a humorous and touching account of his journey through a year of his experience of cancer. In the postscript to the book, he notes that his oncologist told him that "There's no cure. . . . The best we can hope for is a long remission."[64] This does not lead him to despair, though, and he notes that his life had regained some sense of normalcy, even with regular chemotherapy.

Throughout much of the book, Micheli recounts many of the joking comments he made to health professionals during his treatment, adding that much of the humor that he details in his book landed on deaf ears. It is possible, of course, that these various health professionals simply did not know that he was joking or, if they did, that they did not think that his jokes were funny. Alternatively, they could have felt that it would have been unprofessional for them to be laughing while he was dealing with such a serious illness.

In any case, Micheli recounts an example of a nurse who *did* choose to engage him with humor. After receiving eight rounds of chemotherapy, Micheli sat in the doctor's office looking at his latest positron emission tomography (PET) scan. The doctor explained that the tumors, which previously covered his body, were now gone. Still, Micheli writes, this was not reason to rejoice: "The chemo had killed off the cancer in my body, but we all knew I could still—and likely did—have mantle cell percolating in my bone marrow, which, in the absence of the chemo drugs, would soon return lumps and masses throughout my lymph system."[65]

A bone marrow biopsy was needed. "Knowing the level of activity in your marrow," the doctor added, "will help us to gauge how we approach your maintenance chemo over the coming years."[66] The doctor explained that they had to drill into his hip bone to extract the marrow, to which Micheli expressed fear, because of the pain. But the doctor said the pain would be merely a momentary discomfort. When Micheli pressed further, the doctor said that he would be given OxyContin to mitigate the pain. Micheli replied: "OxyContin? I thought you said it would be only a momentary discomfort?"[67] The doctor did not reply.

A week later Micheli returned for the biopsy. He mentioned to the nurse that he did not take the OxyContin because he forgot to fill the prescription. The nurse replied that this should be "memorable."[68] Then they had this interaction:

> What's it [the biopsy] feel like?
> Some people scream.
> Some? What about the others?
> They usually pass out.
> But what does it *feel* like? There's no nerves inside the bone there, so it can't hurt, right?[69]

The nurse then paused, thought about it, laughed, and said: "This one guy, he said it felt like a Harry Potter Dementor sucking his soul out of his ass."[70] Micheli was terrified.

They walked down the hallway into the room for the procedure and had this exchange:

> So, you can pull your pants down and lie on the table.
> Is there, like, a gown I should put on?
> No need.
> No need for you or for me?[71]

The nurse did not reply. Micheli asked when the doctor would arrive. She said in a few minutes. She also explained that his pants needed to be pulled below his buttocks. Micheli notes that he tried to keep the chit chat going despite the awkwardness of the situation. He writes:

> Do you have plans for Christmas? I asked the nurse. I thought about grabbing my cheeks and having my rear end do the talking like Jim Carrey in *Ace Ventura*, but somehow that didn't seem ridiculous enough for the moment. She told me about her plans to visit her grandpa, and from there we moved to swapping dinner recipes, debating whether a smoked or fried turkey was superior, discussing the merits of the new *Star Wars* film, and evaluating the off-season signings of the Washington Nationals. I found myself wondering whether she was making eye contact with me while we chatted [Micheli was positioned

such that his face was to the wall and his back was to the room]. After a while, a lull came to our conversation, and she grew quiet. What are you doing back there? I asked.

Taking a picture.

What?

You haven't seen it? We keep a corkboard in the lab of the best ones. You should feel flattered.[72]

Then the doctor arrived. Micheli goes on to describe the procedure and stated that it did indeed feel like a Harry Potter Dementor sucking his soul out of his ass. He said it is something that he wishes he never has to go through again.

In describing this procedure, he recalls a number of wisecracks that he made to the doctor and the nurse, most of which caused them to laugh or giggle. Also, while he does not comment on it directly, Micheli seems to have really appreciated the flirtatious joke that the nurse made. He comments on sexual matters throughout the book, especially how the experience of cancer and cancer treatment is emasculating, so the nurse's affirmation of his masculinity briefly before a terrifying encounter seemed helpful.

In contrast to *The Diving Bell and the Butterfly, Cancer is Funny* is full of humor, on almost every page Indeed, one sometimes gets the impression as a reader that there is *too much* humor. Yet this is forgivable because Micheli was in—and, to some extent, still is in—such a terrible situation.

This instance of humor regarding the nurse is interesting because some might consider it to be unprofessional in that it is a boundary violation of a sexual nature. However, Micheli does not portray the incident as such, and, again, it seems to have been helpful to him. For this reason I think the nurse's humor should be understood as a boundary crossing rather than a boundary violation. What is the difference? Glen Gabbard suggests that "a boundary crossing is a non-sexual boundary transgression in which the ultimate effect is positive."[73] This boundary crossing was positive for Micheli because the nurse helped Micheli pass the time. After making the joke, she engaged him in conversation with topics that were of interest to him, and she recognized that humor is an important way for Micheli to communicate, either for defensive reasons or other reasons. She compassionately chose to engage him playfully on his terms, tending to his fragile masculinity. By making light of the procedure—by describing it as a Harry Potter Dementor sucking one's soul out of one's ass—she was encouraging him to think of this as something to laugh about, also not unlike the man in Freud's joke who was on his way to the gallows.

Being professional does not mean being humorless. In fact, being professional sometimes requires boundary crossings, to mitigate what would otherwise be a worse harm.

A Pastoral Perspective on Nonmaleficence

For Beauchamp and Childress, nonmaleficence entails avoiding harming patients, populations, and research subjects. As a centric force in bioethics, principlist applications of nonmaleficence tend to focus on, as previously noted, issues such as killing and allowing to die, intending and foreseeing harmful outcomes (e.g., the doctrine of double effect), withholding and withdrawing life-sustaining treatments, extraordinary and ordinary treatments, the underprotection as well as the overprotection of human subjects, and advance directives and surrogate decision-making. While the majority of their discussion focuses on end-of-life issues, Beauchamp and Childress do acknowledge psychosocial harm, and, again, they call for a richer conception of harm. Thus, this is an invitation to offer an eccentric perspective.

My suggestion in this chapter is that with regard to nonmaleficence what is needed is not only richer conceptions of harm but also richer conceptions of the mitigation of harm. Specifically, my suggestion is this: *A pastoral perspective on nonmaleficence considers harm not only in light of physical and psychosocial considerations but also in light of idolatry*. This suggestion, then, is explicitly theological. Indeed, it is grounded in the assumption or observation that human beings have a tendency to make and to worship false gods.

What does idolatry look like with regard to medicine and science? In biomedical contexts idolatry manifests itself when hopes become distorted such that they exacerbate suffering. Humor is one way, though not the only way, of mitigating harms deriving from this idolatry, and the image of the circus clown can be particularly instructive to health professionals and researchers, helping them to reign in their expectations, as it were, bringing the show of modern medicine back to earth.

Further comment is needed with regard to idolatry in this context before the mitigation of idolatry can be appreciated. Idolatry is harmful (and therefore related to nonmaleficence) because idols make promises that they are not capable of fulfilling. Also, to understand what we might call "medical idolatry," some discussion of secularization is helpful. Secularization has many meanings[74] (it should be noted that in recent years many have contested the distinction between the sacred and the secular[75]) but, for my purposes here and without getting too technical or too steeped in secularization theory, I simply want to point out similarities between religion and medicine to draw attention to the existential longings of which they both participate, similarities that have been noted by sociologists and theologians for decades.[76]

In "The Secularization of American Medicine," Roy Branson observes some striking parallels between medicine and religion. Both, he writes, have their "own symbols, values, institutions, and rituals."[77] If, for example, Roman Catholicism has priests who have gone to seminary who learn to lead worship services in churches, medicine likewise has surgeons who have gone to medical school who learn to perform operations in hospitals. Further, whereas priests wear cassocks, doctors wear white coats; whereas priests distribute the sacraments, doctors prescribe medications. To be sure, while doctors also may be compared to other forms of work (e.g., plumbers go to trade schools to learn how to fix sinks in houses), the relationship between medicine and religion is especially fascinating because both religion and medicine make normative moral claims. Branson writes: "Talcott Parsons, who has done as much as anyone to show disease to be not simply a physical condition but a social role, goes so far as to call disease the primary type of deviance in American society. He does so because a person in a diseased condition cannot be effective, cannot achieve."[78]

Physical/medical disease and social/personal sin fit well together. In dentistry, for example, cavities and gingivitis are the result of poor oral health/sin, which is often felt when the dentist asks: "Have you been flossing?" In medicine, too, obesity and diabetes are seen to follow from the sins of gluttony and sloth. Likewise, lung cancer follows from smoking in our moral imaginations, despite the fact that lung cancer presents in many patients who do not smoke.[79] Health professionals are moral judges. Branson writes:

> The fully-robed, impressively self-contained examiner pronounces a verdict on the condition of the diseased. He may grant absolution, saying that the problem is imaginary, or he may absolve the diseased of any guilt for his present condition; none of his past actions have led to his deplorable state. Quite likely the inquisitor points out where there have been some past transgressions contributing to the present turmoil, and prescribes a series of penitential acts by which purity may be regained. The discipline may include the purchase of objects with special powers to assist in achieving full release. If the condition is

> serious a sentence of separation from the healthy may be pronounced. Those untouched by the corruption deserve protection, and the diseased must be encouraged to seek a new life.[80]

Medicine indeed does look a lot like a secularized form of religion.

But, to return to a point that Branson (invoking Parsons) made—namely, that illness is a form of social deviance because it detracts from the demands of work—this insight seems especially American because the sick person cannot fulfill the demands of capitalism. In American society this is a grave sin. In other words, to not work is to be un-American or not fully American, which is to say, deviant. And it is no wonder that in American society "the doctor becomes a priest,"[81] as Branson writes, for doctors are secularly sacralized because they can restore the ill to work. The technology that doctors wield, which is amazing, becomes our new idol.

Near the conclusion of his essay, Branson writes, "Faith in the power of technical reason to save man is dead."[82] On this point, I am not sure he is right. Many persons today with access to health care, perhaps especially in the United States, seem just as devoted to medical technology than ever—it is a "beloved beast."[83] These dollars seem to me to be a sacrifice laid at the altar of Asclepius. And the problem with idols such as medical technology is that they are bound to fail because, as noted, they promise more than they can deliver. Nevertheless, making an idol out of modern medicine is alluring because the promise, if true, would yield considerable happiness: the extra decades of life, the restoration of our youth, the longed-for second chance, the hope of redemption. This distorted religious yearning is understandable. Indeed, it seems few can resist it.

Theologically, what makes these hopes idols? It is the extent to which that they are grand and existential. As Paul Tillich writes, "Idolatry is the elevation of a preliminary concern to ultimacy."[84] For Tillich, faith is having ultimate concern about the ultimate—which is to say, God—and when we put our faith in nonultimate things—in this case, medical technology—we practice idolatry. According to Tillich, idols can be found everywhere: one can make an idol out of faith in ideologies (such as feminism) or in nation states (e.g., patriotism). Indeed, the human capacity for idols is apparently almost endless, which is why the chaplain's perspective, who is always on the lookout for idolatry, is important, and also why the circus clown helpful. A light touch often can be what is healing. What, in the circus of the hospital, is needed is not a lecture on the limits of modern medicine but rather a dose of humility—some humoring of our expectations in addition to our fears.

Caveats

Nonmaleficence, when viewed in light of the circus clown, suggests that health professionals—especially chaplains—can be an agents of perspective via humor so as to mitigate suffering. But caveats are in order. This does not mean that health professionals should become tellers of jokes. This means, rather, that health professionals can share with patients in the humor of their situations. Also, this does not mean engaging in sarcasm, which, from the Greek, literally means tearing of the flesh (what Freud referred to as humor at the expense of others).

I realize that not everyone is able to adopt a humorous attitude, perhaps for reasons of personality or temperament. I also realize that many situations do not call for humor. Indeed, as a part of a scholarly concentration that I direct at McGovern Medical School, there is a journaling component in which medical students write about their clinical encounters. One journal entry in recent years was especially compelling. Genevieve Cruz, a former medical student, has given me her permission to share her experience:

> I've seen pictures of miscarriages in sterile containers and babies that have died prematurely, but I've never seen a 19-week-old baby alive and desperately trying to breath without lungs. She was a perfectly formed human, only 6-inches long, silently gasping for breath.... We couldn't do anything but project our love and sorrow onto this tiny human [being] and be her only moment of human contact in this life. She was too young to have eyes that open but her mouth and chest flailed and her heart pounded visibly through her ribs. The charge nurse look[ed] me in the eye and [said], "I need you to stay here with her; the parents don't want to see her or hold her, so I need you to." Her parents were in too much horror and shock and denial to fathom watching their 19-week-old daughter die—so I was going to. The blur of doctors and nurses across the hall working on mom faded and I stopped listening to what they were whispering.

Cruz continues:

> I held her in my hands as her heart kept right on frantically beating, and for a feeble fleeting moment my brain tried to bargain and reason my way through her surviving. If her heart is still beating, she must be strong.... But then my brain quickly conceded to logic and the science I had been taught. There was nothing functional in her lungs: they

> were closed, thick, and contained no surfactant. Cold hard facts. She continued gasping against a solid organ that would not open. Her heart kept beating, heaving through her ribs. I kept my eyes on her because I didn't want to miss a single beat of her short life. Her fingers and toes were perfectly formed and beautifully delicate. Undeveloped bones caused her body to lie limply . . . so I tried to adjust her, which perhaps only comforted myself. She had no fat or hair on her body and her skin felt left like putty: a tacky layer lacking any keratinization to protect or insulate her. The incubator kept us warm as the minutes kept ticking and I watched her heart keep beating unrelentingly. It felt like hours were passing, yet it would never be enough time to hold her. I could see the flutter of her heart slowing. She had given up trying to gasp and fight against her own body and now lay motionless except for a faint pulsation . . . between her ribs. My eyes stayed on her long after her heart stopped beating.

Situations like these seem profoundly moral, and indeed they are, but they are not primarily about decisions that need to be made or principles to be applied. And there is nothing that humor can do in this moment. All that a chaplain—or anyone—could offer this medical student is presence—not words, but silence, for what words of consolation exist for someone in this moment?

As we struggle for words, sometimes poetry of lament, like the previously cited Sexton poem, can be a healing balm regarding deaths such as these, as Cruz's prose has a certain poetic quality about it. Sometimes suffering can be turned into something beautiful.[85]

Yet, after time has passed, humor can enter again—not regarding particular death (such as the death of this infant) but rather death in general. That is, so-called dark humor *does* have a place in health professional settings; it is not by definition unprofessional. It can be a helpful boundary crossing.

The following anecdote is instructive in this regard. In a class lecture at Princeton Theological Seminary, Robert Dykstra once told a story from his days as a hospital chaplain. (He gave me permission to share this story.) At this hospital it fell to the chaplain to move bodies around after death, from the hospital bed to the morgue, and also to retrieve the bodies when families wished to see the bodies of their loved ones. One day when Dykstra and the other chaplains were orienting a new chaplain they led the new chaplain to the morgue. Another of the chaplains was hiding with a sheet over him in one of the beds where a dead body was presumed to be. And right when the new chaplain was about to pull back the sheet, as he was instructed to do, the hiding chaplain raised out of the bed as though coming back to life. This, of course, gave the new chaplain quite a fright, and laughs were had all around. The prank, while perhaps seeming at the expense of the new chaplain, was actually a way of inviting him into the group as well as a way to ease him into the experience of being a chaplain, dealing with suffering, death, and grief every day. The prank was dark humor, and it was about death, though it also was, in effect, a way of making light of death in general: death as child's play, something to laugh about—though not, to be sure, a particular death, which would be cruel.

A Final Illustration

My thesis in this chapter is not that medical students, residents, physicians, nurses, or other health professionals with technical expertise ought to embrace the image of the circus clown for themselves; this is a pastoral image, appropriate for chaplains to embrace. My thesis, rather, is that the correlation of nonmaleficence and the circus clown reimagines how nonmaleficence can be understood, in that health professionals can mitigate harm not by *being* humorous but by *appreciating* humor. That is, this correlation invites health professionals to take their work seriously but to take themselves less seriously. By taking themselves less seriously, they can help patients to reign in their grand (idolatrous) expectations of modern medicine so that their hopes are realizable.

What might this look like in clinical practice? As in chapter 2, I would like to close with a final illustration involving a patient's perspective. The patient is Donald Capps. He writes:

> Some years ago, I was more-or-less relaxing in a hospital bed waiting to be wheeled off for eye surgery. Another guy was brought into the room in a wheelchair. We shared our stories as to why we were there, then he fell asleep. After a bit, an orderly appeared and said to me, "You the foot?" I said, "No, he's the foot." As they wheeled him out for surgery, I thought about what might have happened if both of us had been asleep, and I had gotten wheeled off for foot surgery. The thought of this was pretty amusing to me at the time, and I couldn't wait to tell the doctor when I arrived in the operation room.[86]

Capps adds: "This was a case of unintentional humor helping me to cope with the anxiety of undergoing surgery. If the orderly had told a joke to the two of us, it may or may not have had the same effect."[87] Capps embodied the humorous attitude toward life that Freud was advocating in his joke about the man headed toward the gallows. As he himself noted, Capps was anxious about his upcoming eye surgery. (Because much of his life was dedicated to reading and writing,[88] the possibility of his work disrupted, perhaps significantly, would have inspired in him dread regarding a fate worse than death.) Thus, this joke, made only to himself at the time, saved him a considerable amount of psychic energy.

Again, however, it is not the place of health professionals to be jokesters, attempting to cheer up patients. The point is, rather, that health professionals would do well to recognize the fact that humor abounds in hospitals, and they can mirror back to patients with a kind smile the humor that patients themselves express. I realize that this is a very mundane suggestion. But subtle interpersonal interactions can help patients transform what might be a living hell into laughing matter, if only briefly. By mirroring back such humor, health professionals can affirm the courageous and rebellious humorous attitudes of patients, which help to mitigate psychosocial harm resulting from existential threats posed by disease and illness.

Also, Capps poked fun at the orderly in a gentle way who, at that moment, was a stand in for modern medicine. His joke brought to light just how unscientific—and how potentially disorganized—hospitals can be. "You the foot?" is hardly a failsafe means of shepherding patients to where they need to go. Moreover, these concerns are not completely unfounded, as there have been cases of patients who have had the wrong limbs amputated and other such surgical mistakes.[89] The hospital is a place not only for amazing feats but also for humor, not unlike the circus. In both places—the hospital and the circus—humor relieves various tensions.

Chapter 2 concluded with a final illustration regarding exemplary behavior of a physician as an expression of what the correlation of that chapter might look like. This chapter, in contrast, concludes with a patient's humorous attitude, also as an expression of what the correlation of this chapter might look like. Capps does not indicate how his physician responded when he shared his humorous thought, but we can hope that this physician supported Capps's own self-mitigation of harm. While there is a modest literature on how physicians and trainees use humor to cope,[90] there is not a comparable body of scholarly work on engaging the humor of patients (Micheli's experience seems to suggest that health professionals could do better in this regard). In any case, exploring this area more deeply and from a variety of perspectives, it seems to me, would contribute to richer conceptions of harm.

4 BENEFICENCE AND THE DIAGNOSTICIAN

In 2013 Daniel Callahan published a controversial essay in the *Hastings Center Report*, titled "Obesity: Chasing an Elusive Epidemic,"[1] in which he offers as one solution to the so-called obesity epidemic in the United States some practical advice on how to encourage overweight persons to lose weight: social shaming. Callahan's argument is interesting and informative, especially as he engages recent public health efforts targeting the epidemic and also because he writes personally about his former smoking habit, how he was quite effectively shamed out of smoking.

Callahan's strategy of social shaming somewhat irritated me as soon as I had read it. Others were irritated as well.[2] As I reflected on why I felt this way, it occurred to me that Callahan, as a philosopher, was not in all likelihood familiar with theological and/or therapeutic literature on shame. What, I wondered, do *philosophers* know about shame, and why should we turn to philosophers regarding questions of personal change? Is not this the realm of therapists? It soon became apparent to me that what I was feeling—more specifically than irritation—was defensiveness because Callahan seemed to be intruding on what I felt to be my intellectual territory. That is to say, while philosophers are good at conceptual analysis, it is the realm of psychologists, pastors, psychotherapists, and other helping professionals to help persons change—*not* philosophers.

Perhaps my feelings are unfair.[3] Maybe Callahan just does a poor job as a philosopher in this particular instance. In any case, Callahan's advice comes across as cold and is likely to be ineffective because he seems controversial for the sake of being controversial. Shame just can't be the answer. Bioethics must have something better to offer.

In contrast to such detached analysis as Callahan's that is somewhat common in bioethics, pastoral theologians, as I have argued in previous chapters, can offer more experience-near accounts of moral questions—and therefore more effective strategies for change—because pastoral theologians draw on the rich traditions of both psychology and theology, as well as other fields and disciplines.

An example of a pastoral theological approach to obesity can be found in the work of Donald Capps, whose work has been featured throughout this book. In a chapter titled "The Inspirational Story" in his book *Living Stories*,[4] Capps focuses on the work of Milton Erickson, who, as noted, was an influential psychiatrist well-known in family therapy circles in the 1960s and 1970s. Capps discusses the case of a woman who had visited Erickson to lose weight. She weighed 180 pounds but wanted to weigh 130 pounds, and her problem was that when she successfully dieted to 130 pounds she would then celebrate her success and subsequently regain the weight. Erickson indicated to her that he could help her but only if she promised to follow his orders, which he said she would not like. She promised to do so. Erickson said: "Your present weight is now 180 pounds. I want you to gain twenty pounds and when you weigh 200 pounds, you may start reducing."[5] The woman begged to be released from the promise but Erickson would not do so and so she gained all of the weight as prescribed. When she was finally permitted to lose weight, she was very happy to do so, and she *did* lose all of the weight, until she weighed 130 pounds. Erickson comments: "Her pattern had been to reduce and gain. I reversed the pattern and made her gain and reduce. And she was very happy with the final results and maintained the weight. She didn't want to, ever again, go through that horrible agony of gaining twenty pounds."[6] I see this as a controversial clinical example of beneficence because Erickson helped her to achieve a goal related to her health (it is controversial in that discussions of women and weight at this historical moment in American culture are gendered[7]—more on this in the following discussion).

Callahan, like Erickson, attempts to address matters of personal change involving weight but a significant difference between the two is that Callahan, as noted, does not engage psychological literature or therapeutic technique in any substantial way. A similarity is that both are manipulative as well as paternalistic (e.g., "doctor knows best" is not far removed from "father knows best"). It seems to me that persons tend to feel enough shame about weight and that what people need are creative ways to get beyond their shame to feel mobilized for change. Capps's use of Erickson does precisely this.

I realize that Erickson's methods might strike the modern reader as authoritarian (and perhaps even patriarchal or antifeminist) as recent trends in therapeutic literature over the past few decades have emphasized more relational understandings of counseling relationships where counselor and counselee co-create meaning and strategies for change.[8] Relatedly, feminist psychotherapist Ellyn Kaschak has considerable experience in working with girls and women who have eating disorders, and in her work she has focused on:

> making visible that which is invisible, self-esteem, reconnecting with other women, identifying multiple meanings and changing meanings in a patriarchal society, and sense of self. . . . Self and context are examined because each defines the other and contributes to the other. Since there is a constant interplay between the two, self and context cannot be separated in feminist therapy.[9]

A weakness, then, of Erickson's approach, from a feminist perspective, is that it likely disregarded contextual factors leading to this woman's request for help in the first place, perhaps suggesting that Erickson was acting in a complicit manner with patriarchal norms that reduce women to adjectives.[10]

However, I am not advocating Erickson per se. My point here is to (i) advocate for psychological theory and therapeutic technique in general, not Erickson in particular, and (ii) emphasize that Callahan could have drawn on psychological and therapeutic literature—even dated literature—that has been shown to have some positive effects. Ideally, it likely would be most helpful to draw on the work of feminist psychologists as well as insights from fat studies when advocating for behavioral change with regard to weight.[11]

Part One: The Principle

The focus of this chapter is on beneficence. I begin in part one by providing an overview of the principle and then offer two classic cases in bioethics that illustrate how it is often understood. One deals with the first heart transplant (to illustrate beneficence at the clinical level) and the other deals with smoking cessation (to illustrate beneficence at the population level). In part two, I move to a discussion of Paul Pruyser's pastoral image of the diagnostician to open up another way of looking at beneficence. In part three, I correlate beneficence with the diagnostician. In the previous chapter, I engaged pathographies as a means of offering experiential inquiry. In this chapter I do so by focusing on a pastoral conversation with a medical resident in my care. I conclude, as in previous chapters, by emphasizing how pastoral aesthetics raises different moral concerns not usually considered by principlism. My argument is that a pastoral perspective on beneficence emphasizes existential well-being.

Beneficence

Beauchamp and Childress suggest that morality not only demands that we should not hurt others—the focus of the previous chapter—but also that we ought to contribute to the welfare of others. Preventive medicine, public health, biomedical research, they observe, are all grounded in beneficence. Beauchamp and Childress distinguish between positive beneficence (where one takes active steps to help another) and utility (where an action, on balance, produces the best overall results), and they note that benevolence is the character virtue associated with the principle of beneficence, which is "a statement of moral obligation."[12]

Beauchamp and Childress ground their understanding of beneficence in reciprocity: "I receive the benefits of society and therefore ought to promote its interests."[13] Applying this logic to physicians, they note that doctors have received the benefits of training (classroom education and clinical teaching) and that some of this education has entailed practicing on patients.[14] Physicians, therefore, owe a large debt to society, to all those who have made the practice of medicine possible: teachers, patients, taxpayers, donors, scientists, administrators, politicians, and so on.[15]

Beauchamp and Childress note that, while some philosophers deny that morality includes positive obligations, they reject this line of thinking, making a distinction between obligatory beneficence and ideal beneficence. They add that extreme personal sacrifice for the sake of others is an ideal—it is not and cannot be required of everyone—and also that there is legitimate debate as to what is obligatory and what is ideal. But, as a baseline as to what is required of everyone, they offer these rules:

1. Protect and defend the rights of others.
2. Prevent harm from occurring to others.
3. Remove conditions that will cause harm to others.
4. Help persons with disabilities.
5. Rescue persons in danger.[16]

They distinguish nonmaleficence from beneficence in these ways:

> Rules of nonmaleficence (1) are negative prohibitions of action, (2) must be followed impartially, and (3) provide moral reasons for legal prohibitions of certain forms of conduct. By contrast, rules of beneficence (1) present positive requirements of action, (2) need

> not always be followed impartially, and (3) generally do not provide reasons for legal punishment when agents fail to abide by them.[17]

Further, they distinguish between general and specific beneficence. Specific beneficence entails, for example, moral obligations parents have to children. Thus, specific beneficence is relational and contextual. But general beneficence, as the term implies, is broader, applying to all people (i.e., we have obligations not only to our own family but also to families all over the world) and perhaps even to all beings (i.e., beyond our own species). Beauchamp and Childress note that Peter Singer is well known for his widening of the moral circle[18] to include animals[19] (Singer also has written extensively on the topic of global poverty, arguing that geographical distance is an arbitrary moral consideration when contemplating aiding others—more on this in the next chapter).[20]

Against those who think that morality does not require positive action on behalf of others, Beauchamp and Childress discuss a landmark legal case in psychiatric ethics, the *Tarasoff* case. This case involved a situation in which a therapist learned of his patient's intention to kill a specific woman (the patient's love interest). While the therapist did notify the police, he did not notify the woman, and the patient later murdered the woman. Beauchamp and Childress write "Only a remarkably narrow account of moral obligation would assert that the psychiatrist is under no obligation to protect the woman by contacting her or the police or both."[21] They add: "If morality does not demand this much beneficence, it is difficult to see how morality imposes any positive obligations at all."[22]

After this general discussion of beneficence, Beauchamp and Childress move on to discuss specific issues in bioethics. One issue is expanded access and compassionate use programs. These programs are intended to give patients who want access to investigational products that are not yet approved. The use of azidothymidine (AZT) during the human immunodeficiency virus/acquired immunodeficiency syndrome (HIV/AIDS) epidemic in the United States, for example, is a case in point, because in the 1980s the epidemic was considered to be fatal (so activists reasonably felt that a placebo-controlled trial was cruel because this meant withholding, for the sake of science, a potentially life-saving drug to otherwise dying patients).[23] But Beauchamp and Childress note that a common problem with these programs is that they often increase risk without increasing benefits at the individual level.[24] Today, a related problem is therapeutic misconception, when patients enroll in a research protocol believing that they will benefit from experimental therapy when it is almost certain that they will not.

Continued access programs raise related problems. Here the issue is that, if an experimental therapy is found to be effective, to what extent should research participants be given continued access to the therapy after the research study is completed? It would seem unfair to deny former research participants of effective treatment after they put themselves at risk. But what if researchers cannot afford to do so?

Another issue Beauchamp and Childress discuss at considerable length is the issue of paternalism, as it demonstrates common conflicts between beneficence and respect for autonomy. Paternalism refers to rule by a father or parent. With regard to medicine, paternalism is treating a patient as though he or she were a child, making decisions for them. Beauchamp and Childress define paternalism in bioethics as "*the intentional overriding of one person's preferences or actions by another person, where the person who overrides justifies this action by appeal to the goal of benefiting or of preventing or mitigating harm to the person whose preferences or actions are overridden.*"[25] Examples include performing cardiopulmonary resuscitation (CPR) on an unconscious patient who has signed a do not resuscitate (DNR) order to save her or his life, involuntarily committing a patient to a psychiatric hospital during acute psychosis, and withholding medical information from a patient that a physician feels may diminish the patient's hope. Paternalism also can be applied toward communities, as when city officials infuse water with fluoride against the wishes of some members of the community. It is easy to see, therefore, how beneficence can conflict with respect for autonomy.

Beauchamp and Childress make a distinction between soft and hard paternalism. The former is when a physician intervenes to prevent nonvoluntary conduct (e.g., when a patient is making poor decisions, perhaps due to an acute depression, that otherwise he or she likely would not make). The latter is when a physician overrides some ill-advised choice by a patient despite the fact that the patient does understand the risks and the consequences of his or her decision (e.g., when an adult Jehovah's Witness refuses a routine blood transfusion, knowingly endangering his or her own life). Passive paternalism is when a patient's request is ignored because it is believed to be inappropriate (e.g., when a patient requests elective amputation of a healthy limb[26] or tubal ligation at a young age). Refusing to treat on the grounds of futility—also a form of passive paternalism—is sometimes practiced (cf. chapter 3).

Beauchamp and Childress also discuss surrogate decision-making, an issue closely related to respect for autonomy. When patients suffer from a stroke, Parkinson's disease, or Alzheimer's disease, sometimes they need others to make decisions for them. There are different ways of thinking about how best to make these decisions. Beauchamp and Childress discuss three: the substituted judgement standard, the pure autonomy standard, and the best interests standard. The substituted judgement standard requires a surrogate "to make the decision the incompetent person would have made if competent."[27] The pure autonomy standard rests on prior statements made by persons when they were competent, as in an advance directive, though also in less formal statements. The best interests standard is useful when the person's preferences simply are not known. It is a decision made on probable quality-of-life.

In terms of health policy, Beauchamp and Childress discuss cost-effective analysis, cost–benefit analysis, and risk–benefit analysis. Cost refers to the use of resources to bring about a desired outcome. Benefit is usually understood to be a positive outcome, though it can sometimes be understood as the avoidance of a harm. And risk refers to the chance of a harmful outcome or effect. Policy recommendations are based on assessments of various procedures and products. An interesting example that they discuss in this regard is breast implants in healthy young women. They note that in 2006 it was found that, while there are "frequent local complications and adverse outcomes" as a result of these procedures, the Food and Drug Administration (FDA) did not propose a ban on these procedures because it was "determined that their benefits and risks are 'sufficiently well understood for women to make informed decisions about their use.' "[28] Thus, the FDA took an antipaternalistic stance with regard to breast implants because it is difficult to quantify the perceived benefit by women of this procedure and women do tend to report significant levels of happiness after receiving breast implants. While these happiness levels appear to remain stable over time,[29] the known risks are real and remain.

Beauchamp and Childress close the chapter by discussing quality-of-life. A key term in health policy is quality-adjusted life years (QALY), which is defined as "a measure of health outcome which looks at both length of life and quality-of-life. QALYs are calculated by estimating the years of life remaining for a patient following a particular care pathway and weighting each year with a quality-of-life score."[30] Beauchamp and Childress note that there are ethical values or commitments (e.g., utilitarianism) inherent in this way of thinking, and prejudices or biases as well. Indeed, age discrimination is embedded in this way of thinking.

Beauchamp and Childress's interpretation of beneficence may be summarized as follows. They describe two aspects of beneficence: positive beneficence (which focuses on providing benefits to others) and utility (which focuses on attempting to achieve the best overall results). They also make a distinction between obligations and ideals. Paternalism is sometimes justified, they argue, though other principles (such as respect for autonomy) set limits on paternalism. With regard to surrogate decision-making, in most cases what is known about a patient's preferences should be respected, though sometimes what is in the patient's best interests, from a medical standpoint, can override patient preferences. Formal techniques of analysis to assess risks and benefits are useful, though considerations of justice may set limits on calculations of utility.

To do good for persons and groups, some kind of assessment about what is in their best interests is needed, as determined by clinical judgement and scientific data. This is why beneficence is closely related to paternalism. Laypersons, to a great extent, do not have or understand this knowledge. Therefore, this principle is specified by experts. While sometimes what beneficence indicates is straightforward (e.g., school-age children should receive certain vaccinations[31]), other times what beneficence indicates is unclear. Making subjective assessments about a person's desired quality-of-life, for example, is difficult, as is ascertaining whether to give health or liberty more weight while making decisions on behalf of a community, because scientific facts and moral values can become conflated, muddled, and confused. Two illustrations follow to demonstrate what considerations of beneficence look like in practice.

An Illustration: The First Heart Transplant

The first surgeon to do a heart transplant was Christiaan Barnard. Born in South Africa, Barnard received his medical degree in 1953 and later traveled to the United States for a two-year fellowship (from 1956 to 1958) at the University of Minnesota Medical School, where he studied with Owen Wangansteen. He also spent a week in Houston, Texas, learning from Michael DeBakey and Denton Cooley. In 1958, after having received a doctorate in surgery, he returned to South Africa to serve as the director of research at the University of Cape Town Medical School. He continued making trips abroad to stay current with the latest surgical techniques.[32]

Gregory Pence writes that the "first heart transplant was not performed, as might have been expected, at a prestigious center of medical research; it took place at an obscure hospital in Cape Town, South Africa, called Groote Schuur."[33] He notes that in 1966 the surgical consensus was that a heart transplant would not be, from a strictly technical point of view, that difficult, but it was unknown how to keep the human body from rejecting a new heart, so a heart transplant therefore had not been attempted yet. It was viewed as too dangerous.

The patient in need of the heart transplant was Louis Washkansky. At the age of fifty-five, he was suffering from diabetes, coronary artery disease, and congestive heart failure. In 1966 he was expected to live for only a month or two more, but he kept on living, though his condition continued to worsen. The donor was a twenty-five-year-old woman, Denise Darvall, who was declared brain-dead after an automobile accident. Prior to the operation, Barnard said to Washkansky, "We can put a normal heart into you, after taking out your heart that's no longer good, and there's a chance you can get back to normal life."[34]

The operation was on December 3, 1967, and the removal of the hearts and the transplanting of one was not incredibly difficult—just as expected. But what was unclear was whether the new heart would start beating and whether the body would accept it. Pence writes: "According to United Press International (UPI), the transplanted heart began to beat after Barnard shocked it slightly, whereupon Barnard gasped, 'Christ, it's going to work!' "[35]

Pence notes that Washkansky's new heart eventually started beating correctly, after it had stopped briefly, and that it also took some time to take over from the heart–lung machine. Remarkably, Washkansky regained consciousness on the same day of his operation, and he was able to eat about two days later. But the next five days were poor, followed by five good days, which led to his rapid decline and death, after having lived eighteen days postsurgery. The problem was, also just as others had expected, that his body rejected the transplanted heart. After his death, it was found that lobar pneumonia had destroyed his lungs, even while, Pence writes, "the heart itself and Barnard's surgery were perfect."[36] The response to Barnard's operation was mixed. Many felt that the attempt was made too soon, while others, such as DeBakey, stated that "Barnard had broken through a medical barrier."[37]

Pence suggests that one of the most important ethical issues raised by this case is quality-of-life—one of the key considerations of beneficence, as previously noted. What, exactly, would constitute a "successful" heart transplant for Washkansky? Would it be simply a successful transplant? Or would it be something more, such as enabling him to live for years? Pence also notes that informed consent was an issue in this case: Did Washkansky really know how minimal his chances of survival were and how painful his death was almost certain to be? This seems unlikely, for while he was dying he refused further medical treatment, but Barnard forced it on him anyway. The heart transplant inflicted a great deal of harm on Washkansky for very little gain. This was a violation of nonmaleficence.

But perhaps the surgery could be viewed in light of medical progress and that Washkansky's death led to the saving of many more lives in the future—thus, a justification based on utility (beneficence)—but this justification seems weak as well, given that Washkansky died exactly for the reasons other surgeons were reluctant to do the surgery. To frame this case in light of beneficence—in contrast to nonmaleficence—it was a failed attempt to rescue (in any meaningful way) a man in danger, whose only possibility of living for a substantial amount of time would be with a new heart. Washkansky was given a chance to live, and he wanted to take it.

An Illustration: The Ethics of Smoking Cessation Programs

Beneficence, as noted, also often has policy implications. Governments make rules and regulations that limit liberty for the public good. A classic illustration of this are the efforts of public health professionals to persuade people to refrain from smoking.

In "No Smoking: The Ethical Issues," Robert Goodin notes that there is a long philosophical tradition that defends the view that "it is not the place of society to stop us from doing things that will harm no one but ourselves."[38] On the surface, this line of thinking would seem to apply to smoking: If people want to harm themselves by ingesting toxins, why stop them? But on closer inspection, Goodin argues, this view is difficult to hold because it is well known now that secondhand smoke does harm others, which is why there are widespread restrictions on smoking in public places (e.g., restaurants, offices, bars, airplanes, etc.).

Also, it is not clear that smokers both knowingly and voluntarily accept the risks of smoking because in the past tobacco companies distributed conflicting information regarding the health effects of smoking,[39] sowing confusion in the general public. Thus, people were not adequately informed about their choices. Relatedly, Goodin notes that studies have shown that many adult smokers began smoking when they were teenagers—before the legal age of consent—so by the time that they became old enough to consent, they were already addicted. This, too, is not adequate consent. Furthermore, Goodin concedes that while people can, and do, quit smoking, most smokers do not, which suggests that expecting smokers to quit may be unreasonable because it is too hard to do so.

While people may voluntarily consent when they smoke their first cigarette, they do not voluntarily *continue* smoking, because they are addicted. This is why, Goodin argues, there needs to be strong disincentives in place to prevent people from beginning to smoke in the first place. These disincentives include placing warnings on packages of cigarettes, running ad campaigns that educate the public about the hazards of smoking, placing high taxes on the sale of tobacco, banning smoking from public places, and fining those who sell tobacco to minors.

Goodin also addresses the social costs of smoking, noting its disutility: "We do not leave it to the discretion of customers, however well-informed, whether or not to drink grossly polluted water, ingest grossly contaminated foods, or inject grossly dangerous drugs."[40] He adds that public health actions are justified when, for example, contagious diseases risk threatening a population, both in terms of health effects and in terms of financial cost. Regarding cost, if a particular cohort (such as smokers) increase health care spending for the whole group, then this group should be required to pay a premium to offset these costs to the group—another disincentive. All of these disincentives are paternalistic, but they are in place both to protect the health of individuals and the health of society. To view these efforts in light of beneficence, they are aimed at actively preventing harm from occurring to others.

Part Two: The Image

Having provided an overview of beneficence, as well as illustrations of it at both the clinical and population levels, I now want to turn to the diagnostician to set the stage for offering a pastoral perspective on beneficence.

The Diagnostician

Pruyser was a clinical psychologist associated with the Menninger Clinic when it was in Topeka, Kansas, and he was very close with Karl Menninger, a prominent psychiatrist in the United States in the twentieth century.[41] In "The Diagnostician" Pruyser argues for, as the title suggests, the image of the diagnostician as one for pastors He notes that ministers are unlikely to think of themselves in this way because the dominant image for pastors is the shepherd and the prevailing image for congregations is sheep.[42] However, when sheep are in need of help, Pruyser reasons, they would be normally taken to a veterinarian—that is, a health professional. He elaborates:

> If "shepherd" and "sheep" are metaphors for people, the pastor can have his ill folk diagnosed by a medical doctor or a psychiatrist, who are alleged to know far more than he does about sizing up human beings when they complain of physical and mental problems. The pastor will gladly help his people in trouble, but he surely will not consider himself an expert in diagnosis.[43]

"But," Pruyser adds, "what if some people have a desire to be assessed, evaluated, diagnosed by their pastors?"[44] He continues:

> What if certain persons want to make an honest assessment of themselves, and turn to their pastors for expert help in making a diagnosis of their troubles, their foibles, their stance in life, their troublesome, puzzlesome, or wayward selves? What if they want precisely their pastors, rather than some other specialists, to guide them in their search for a self-diagnosis? What if they want to place themselves in a pastoral theological rather than a medical, psychiatric, legal, or social perspective? What if they want to be in several professional hands at one and the same time?[45]

Pruyser's main argument is that that pastors have their own specialized form of knowledge that they should not abandon in favor of secular (often psychological) language and categories.

Why do persons turn to their pastors first for help? Pruyser offers several possibilities: accessibility, economics, and trust. It is easier to drop in to see pastors unannounced and to visit with them at no charge. Parishioners also often have a relationship with their pastor, making them prone to trusting them. Still, Pruyser believes that people go to pastors for deeper reasons than these. He thinks that people often are seeking a pastoral perspective even if they cannot articulate what that means: "They may not know how to phrase their wish, hoping that their pastor will make the first move in that direction by offering the right words or making the pertinent allusions."[46] He continues:

> Some may simply wish to pray, if only the pastor would offer to do so. Some may wish to be blessed, if only their pastor would be so inclined. Others may wish to be decisively confronted with their failings or disloyalties, if only their pastor had the forthrightness to do so. What parishioners expect from their pastor emerges from a complicated mixture of hopes, fears, fantasies, ambivalent feelings, and reality

> testing, all charged with a double set of numinous values: on the one hand those inherent in religion and the transcendent, on the other hand the numinosity of parental power and grandeur experienced in childhood.[47]

He adds: "Pastors are transference figures par excellence, not necessarily by what they are as persons but by the projections of those who seek their counsel."[48]

What would a pastor's diagnosis look like? Pruyser suggests that "his state of grace, his despair, his deep or shaken loyalty, his tenets or disbeliefs, his grounds for hope, if any, his rebelliousness or his tendency to deny any responsibility" might serve as diagnostic categories.[49] These seem like a good starting point when correlating beneficence and the diagnostician.

Part Three: Correlation of Principle and Image

This chapter is experientially-grounded by focusing on the case of Atlas (not his real name). Atlas approached me precisely because he wanted his life to be seen in pastoral perspective. He gave me permission to tell his story. In fact, he suggested that I do so, and he requested me to be "unflichingly true."

Because pastoral counseling is an accredited enterprise,[50] I will refer to my various encounters with Atlas simply as pastoral conversation. Also, while pastoral counseling, like secular psychotherapy, is paid, my conversations with Atlas were at no cost. I am an ordained minister in the Presbyterian Church (U.S.A.), and I serve as volunteer chaplain for the United Campus Ministries of Greater Houston, providing pastoral care for students and residents in the Texas Medical Center as a part of this unpaid ministry.

In terms of theology, psychology, and therapy, I turn to Capps's engagement with reframing literature to shed light on Atlas's experience. The diagnostician fits nicely with the method of reframing in that various reframing techniques are sometimes viewed with suspicion because they are paternalistic, not unlike traditional applications of beneficence in bioethics.

A Pastoral Perspective on Beneficence

For Beauchamp and Childress beneficence is about taking active steps to help others as well as seeking to achieve the best overall results. Applying this principle often entails thinking through the tension between acting paternalistically toward versus respecting the autonomy of others. Usually the weighing, balancing, and specifying of beneficence rests heavily on data. As a centric force in bioethics, principlist applications of beneficence tend to focus on issues such as, as previously noted, expanded and continued access in research, surrogate decision-making, and quality-of-life assessments.

I suggest that, as an eccentric force in bioethics, a pastoral perspective on beneficence also focuses on doing good for others, and it, too, can be paternalistic. But what it adds that is distinctive, specifically, can be put this way: *A pastoral perspective on beneficence places an emphasis on existential well-being as influenced by the caregiver.* Placing an emphasis on existential well-being is different from, though related to, medical and/or psychological well-being, in that existential well-being attends to the soul, which is different from the self, the mind, the brain, and so on.[51] And because these interventions are influenced by the pastoral caregiver, they can be paternalistic.

The Case of Atlas

Atlas is married with one child, a son. He took a seminar that I offer for medical students, titled Pathographies of Mental Illness. The course was inspired by one that I took in seminary, taught by Capps, titled the Minister and Mental Illness,[52] which is organized by mental illness.

The final paper that Atlas wrote for the course was titled "Atlas Unshrugged." A figure from Greek mythology, Atlas holds up the sky. In paintings and sculptures, he is often depicted with the world on his shoulders. This, for good reason, is how this man felt when he came to see me.

After the class had ended, Atlas asked me if he could see me for pastoral counseling. He explained to me that he was seeing a psychologist already but that he felt that the psychologist did not address his spiritual needs adequately. Atlas enjoys deep things (such as *Hamlet* as well as the writings of C. G. Jung) very much, and he was curious about what light pastoral counseling could shed on his life.

During our first several meetings as well as in his course paper, Atlas slowly revealed his various sufferings and losses to me. His brother, who for years suffered from back pain, was diagnosed with a rare form of cancer. As he was dying, he cried out to Atlas to find a way to stop the pain, leaving Atlas disillusioned with mainstream medical practice with regard to pain management. Far too many patients suffer needlessly, Atlas has witnessed, in part because doctors are afraid of their dying patients becoming addicted to pain medication. Atlas saw his brother suffer too much for no reason.

As his brother was undergoing treatment related to his cancer, his dad also was suffering from back pain. He was found to have this rare form of cancer as well. On the day of his brother's death, Atlas had to drive his father to a hospital. While still grieving the death of his brother, Atlas now was required to help care for his father—and also to try to continue medical school. His father had many ups and downs, many close calls, but eventually stabilized after some months, with intermittent periods of crises and hospitalizations, which continue to this day. Atlas moved from one crisis to the next, through no fault of his own. It was just the hand that life had dealt him.

But Atlas was getting tired of playing this hand, especially when he began experiencing acute back pain himself. The pain got so bad that he feared that his cancer diagnosis was next. Fortunately, that did not happen. Nevertheless, Atlas lives in a state of chronic pain. Each morning, because he is exhausted from not sleeping due to the pain, he drinks several caffeinated sodas (he does not like the taste of coffee).

At work Atlas is not able to stand for long periods of time, so he moves through the hospital in a wheelchair. While walking, he uses a cane. Perhaps for a mixture of all of these reasons, and more, he also suffers from periods of sadness.

So Atlas has dealt with and continues to deal with a lot: chronic back pain, grief concerning the death of his brother, and anticipated grief and anxiety concerning the death of his father. Just when it seemed as though things could not get worse, they did.

One day the Federal Bureau of Investigation (FBI) appeared at his house while he was on a clinical rotation. The FBI informed his wife that Atlas was under arrest for the possession and distribution of child pornography. When he found out, Atlas was taken completely by surprise, for he knew that this was all a misunderstanding. He also knew that this still would be a very stressful, anxiety-provoking, and time-consuming process of setting the record straight. Atlas had nothing to do with child pornography.

It did turn out to be a misunderstanding. The FBI ascertained that it was Atlas's teenage son who was the true source of their investigation. Atlas's son was accused of creating, possessing, and distributing child pornography. He was arrested and a judge ruled that, because of the severity of the crime—he was accused of sexually abusing a child—he was to be tried as an adult. Atlas cashed out all of his savings and his 401(k), and he borrowed all of the money that he could from friends and family for legal fees to defend his son.

Atlas's son did not deny what he had done. His defense was that he did what he did because he was abused when he was a child by a family member. The jury did not find this defense compelling. Atlas's son was found guilty.

Then the worst thing happened. In prison, Atlas's son attempted suicide. He was acting bizarrely as well. Talking with his son on the phone and also visiting with him in prison, Atlas began to suspect his son suffered from a mental disorder. A psychiatrist later confirmed a particular diagnosis. It is this aspect of Atlas's suffering—his son's mental illness—about which he feels most helpless.

Atlas continues to care for his son, but this is difficult because his son is moved all across the state to various prisons on a regular basis. Atlas wonders what it means to be a father now and how he can care for his son. His son has proven to be remarkably resilient, being able to make it through months of solitary confinement. Still, because of inadequate access to mental health care in the prison system, his son has had several relapses as well as many episodes of cutting. While cutting should not always be understood as a suicide attempt, it is nevertheless concerning—more weight on Atlas's shoulders. Recently Atlas explained to me that his son "cut himself over a 100 times with a razor and ended up in segregation (suicide cell) for 5 days. They had to pepper spray him to get him to stop. Yesterday was my day off and I spoke at length with him for the first time since it happened. I was able to talk him off the ledge."[53] So this is Atlas's situation: a living hell.

What is remarkable about Atlas is how high functioning he is. Not only was he able to complete medical school under circumstances in which most people could not, but also he was able to complete a demanding residency. It is striking how likable Atlas is. He does not come across as depressed or even bitter. Rather, he comes across as calm and gentle. He is quick to laugh and to find humor in even dark matters, especially concerning his own suffering. Though he is quick to laugh, he explains that, during periods of despair that he sometimes expereinces, he finds no joy in anything, which is worse, he says, than any physical pain he has ever experienced, even his back pain.

Reframing

In *Reframing: A New Method in Pastoral Care*, Capps writes not for pastoral care specialists (e.g., pastoral counselors), because they are familiar with reframing techniques, but for pastors.[54] As many health care professionals—for example, doctors, nurses, dentists, and so on—do not have much exposure to counseling techniques, certainly not more so than pastors, what Capps writes for pastors is therefore helpful for health care professionals.

Capps bases his discussion on a book by Paul Watzlawick, John Weakland, and Richard Fisch, titled *Change: Principles of Problem Formation and Problem Resolution*.[55] The method of reframing was developed at the Brief Therapy Center of the Mental Research Institute in Palo Alto, California. In *Change*, Watzlawick, Weakland, and Fisch contend that there are two kinds of change: first-order change and second-order change. First-order change is a change within a given system that does not change the system. Second-order change changes the system. As an example of first-order change, they provide this example: "A drinker provokes criticism and surveillance of his drinking by his wife. As she complains and attempts to 'protect' him from alcohol, his drinking increases, which, in turn, brings about an increase in her criticism, etc."[56] The problem was the fact that the husband was drinking too much and the solution, attempted at the first-order level, was to survey his drinking. However, this approach only made matters worse.

What does a second-order change look like? Capps offers this example of second-order change as a typical employment of reframing by a therapist:

> A therapist is working with a family and the father says, "Nobody in this family has ever supported me by taking care of me. I always have to do it all by myself." . . . To this the therapist responds, "Thank God!" The father, of course, expected some kind of supporting comment like, "Oh, that's really too bad. Maybe we can make changes in the family." Instead, the father has organized his life in such a way that no one in his family feels it necessary to take care of him—a very positive achievement.[57]

Thus, second-order change challenges the structure or rules of what is perceived to be the problem, creating new dynamics and new possibilities for relating.

But what about an example relating to alcohol, since the example of the first-order change previously offered failed? And what about an example that is relevant to health professionals? In *Living Stories*, Capps offers an example that addresses both of these questions. It is another case from Erickson.[58] (If the previous Erickson case in this chapter regarding helping a woman to lose weight was offensive, in part because it involved a man paternalistically interacting with a woman, this case involves a man interacting paternalistically with a man.) Here is the case:

> A medically retired policeman told me, "I have emphysema, high blood pressure, and, as you can see, I am grossly overweight. I drink too much. I eat too much. I want a job but my emphysema and high blood pressure prevent that. I would like to cut down on my smoking. I'd like to get rid of it. I'd like to quit drinking about a fifth of whiskey a day and I'd like to eat sensibly."[59]

Erickson asked about the man's daily habits with regard to eating, drinking, and smoking. The man explained that there was a grocery store close to him and that he bought his meals and cigarettes there, and he could buy his alcohol nearby as well. After listening to this, Erickson gave the man these instructions:

> Walk across town to buy your [cigarettes]. That will start to get you into shape. As for your groceries, don't shop at the handy grocery around the corner. Go to a grocery a half-mile or a mile away and buy just enough for each meal. That means three nice walks a day. As for your liquor, you can drink all you want to. Take your first drink at a bar at least a mile away. If you want a second drink, find another bar at least a mile away. If you want a third, find another bar a mile away.[60]

The man stormed out of his office in anger. However, a month later, a new referral presented in Erickson's office, referred to him by the police officer, saying that the police officer "said you are the one psychiatrist who knows what he is doing."[61] Unlike the failed attempt at a first-order change involving alcohol previously noted, Erickson surprised this man with his advice—specifically because alcohol and tobacco were not taken away from him. A commentator on this case noted that "Erickson recognized that he was dealing with a man who had a long history of carrying out orders [because he was a police officer]. Therefore, he gives him orders with the expectation that the man will carry them out. This is an important example of meeting the patient in his frame of reference."[62]

The Technique of Relabeling

In *Reframing*, Capps discusses many therapeutic techniques, including, but not limited to, dereflection, confusion, advertising instead of concealing, offering the illusion of alternatives, providing a worse alternative, relabeling, preempting, prescription, and surrender. The technique presented in the following discussion is that of relabeling because it is what I used with Atlas.

Relabeling, as the term implies, entails giving a different label to behaviors, attitudes, or situations than that which the counselee gives to them. Relabeling also is supposed to offer a more accurate description. It is not a trick or a gimmick. To illustrate this technique, Capps discusses a counseling session of Mr. and Mrs. Blackright. They have been seeing their pastor for marriage counseling, during which they discuss a recent incident of Mr. Blackright spilling orange juice on the floor. Here is the exchange among the three:

PASTOR: What happened [after he spilled it]?
MRS. B: I came charging in, yelled at him to be more careful, and then cleaned up the mess.
PASTOR: Why did *you* clean it up?
MRS. B: I knew he'd take hours to get around to it, and he'd make another mess in cleaning up that one!
PASTOR: How did you feel about her cleaning up the mess?
MR. B: She's a perfectionist! Always after me to do something! I can never do anything well enough to please her! She wouldn't have liked the way I cleaned up the floor.
PASTOR: Anything else?
MR. B: [With a sly smile] Well, I suppose I knew that if I waited a little while she'd do it.[63]

Capps notes that both partners label each other—messy and perfectionist—though neither label is accurate, at least in this situation. Capps writes:

> On the basis of this episode, a more accurate label for Mr. Blackright would be *dependent*, since he acts toward his wife like a little boy who relies on his mother to set things right, and complains that she expects too much from him. And Mrs. Blackright may be described as a person who *dominates* her husband, insisting on doing things for him which he could easily do for himself.[64]

Capps adds that the advantage of these labels, in contrast to the labels of messy and perfectionist, imply that change is possible, because while messy and perfectionist are personality traits (and therefore hard to change) dependent and dominating are relational descriptions (and therefore subject to change). "When pastors relabel the behavior of individuals, of groups, or of the congregation as a whole," Capps continues, "they should choose words to describe the present situation as the effect of mutable rather than immutable factors so as to reinforce the conviction that desirable change is quite possible."[65]

Relabeling Atlas's Experiences

For any Christian familiar with the Bible, Atlas's suffering recalls the story of Job, which Atlas himself brought up in our sessions. The story of Job, briefly, is as follows.[66]

Job, an upright man, has prospered in life because he has obeyed God, just as the Torah indicates blessings for obedience and curses for disobedience (see Deuteronomy 28). But Satan[67] provokes God by saying: "Does Job fear [You] for nothing? Have You not put a fence around him and his house and all that he has, on every side? You have blessed the work of his hands, and his possessions have increased in the land. But stretch out Your hand now, and touch all that he has, and he will curse You to Your face" (Job 1:9-11). God then puts Job to a number of tests, allowing many terrible things to happen to Job. Job loses his wealth, his children die, and his health deteriorates. Job's friends attempt to comfort him but to no avail. Angry and desperate, Job confronts God. God responds by stating that Job has no right to question God's authority. The book ends, however, with God restoring Job's health and wealth and by giving new children to him.

There is much more to the story than this, of course. Capps, for example, creatively reads the Book of Job in light of various counseling techniques, arguing that God is able to achieve second-order change with Job via reframing techniques.[68] But this is the basic arc of the narrative, about which Atlas was familiar.

Atlas said to me that he felt that he really could not endorse the story of Job. Something seemed right about the story, but something seemed off as well. The sort of happy ending did not work for him because, after all, Job's original children were still dead—the ending is not *that* happy. Moreover, God never explained to Job why he was suffering or why God would let Godself be influenced by Satan.

I agreed with Atlas's assessment. And I told him so. Disagreeing or debating with him, of course, would not be helpful, placing us in adversarial roles. Atlas felt abandoned by God (in effect, worse than Job, because Atlas had not received any happy ending from God, whereas Job did). What Atlas needed was my support and—more importantly—a more complex understanding of God, an image of God that fit more closely with his experience. He intuited that the Book of Job could give him this, but he wasn't sure how. His previous attempts at explaining Job's suffering only left him feeling dissatisfied with the narrative.

I then told Atlas about what some biblical scholars have written about the Book of Job. Specifically, I mentioned that biblical scholars have observed that the majority of the Book of Job is written in poetry, while the beginning and the end are written in prose, leading scholars to conclude that the Book of Job probably had different authors and was written at different times likely with different motives and concerns. I also pointed out that many scholars think that the poetry portions of Job are older than the prose sections and that the prose beginning and end was intended to frame the narrative in a certain way. I further pointed out that the bet between God and Satan, as well as the ending, was a part of the prose (and therefore was added later) because Job's lament was probably too radical for some faith communities. If the poetry section were left to stand on its own, Job's suffering has no explanation. Moreover, in the poetry section, Job receives no restoration after God scolds Job for questioning God's authority.[69] Suffering is left to be a mystery. In effect, by telling Atlas about some conclusions about the Book of Job by biblical scholars, the narrative was relabeled as *mystery*, whereas previously it was labeled by Atlas as *unsatisfying*.

With regard to reframing, Atlas reflected on the Book of Job for many years, never able to find a compelling interpretation. This is because he was viewing it through the same frame—the frame of the narrative itself. His various attempts to engage the Book of Job by reflecting on the narrative itself may be viewed as attempts of first-order change. But by offering Atlas a different frame—the frame of biblical scholarship—the meaning of the Book of Job changed. It was no longer about *explaining* suffering but instead it was about *expressing* suffering. And Atlas felt that the existential implications of these critical readings of the Book of Job were congruent with his own experience, for he knew that he did nothing to deserve all of the suffering that he had received, and he also knew that there would not be some kind of an easy happy ending. His son probably will remain in prison for decades to come, his chronic pain likely will continue, and sadness as well as despair will always be a possibility. Still, by affirming God's presence in this suffering was grounds for hope for Atlas, for though suffering is a mystery, there is still order. Paradox and mystery imply that change is possible. Why? Because not having the answers is sometimes more liberating than having them. This is second-order change.

Relatedly, Capps observes that while God does not explain Job's suffering, or apologize for it, God points out paradoxical features of the natural world (see, e.g., Job 39:13–18, where the ostrich is portrayed as both stupid and majestic), and Capps writes:

> In noting the paradoxical nature of the universe, God indirectly addressed Job's situation. If the world itself is inherently paradoxical, then it should not be surprising that a blameless man suffers and a wicked man goes to his grave happy and contented. If the world were rationally ordered, this would not happen. But the order of the world is paradox, which is not disorder or sheer chaos, but a curious kind of order.[70]

Profound suffering in this life just does not have an answer.[71] A biblical affirmation of this existential truth, however dark, paradoxically provides hope, simply by being a part of the canon. Not a resolution of suffering, but a witnessing of the mystery of life and a hope that meaning will arise out of or in spite of suffering.[72]

During a different session, Atlas talked about the various weights in his life along with a new one. A family member who has served in the military suffers from posttraumatic stress disorder (PTSD) and alcoholism. After an especially severe drinking binge, Atlas was required to help this family member in finding treatment for his addiction. Reflecting on his life, Atlas expressed to me a fantasy in which he ran away to Africa, away from all of his problems. This led to my asking about his marriage because I feared that he might be entertaining the idea of leaving his wife, probably the most stable force in his life. Surprised by my question, he reported that his wife had expressed concern about their relationship the previous night. In response to her, Atlas explained that he just had no energy for the relationship right now. I began wondering if the weight was too much for Atlas to bear. I asked him, "Is there a way that you can set limits on the demands that other people make on you?" He said that this was really hard because he always was going to help his son as well as other family members. Indeed, how could he not?

On another occasion, Atlas requested to see me immediately because he was feeling overwhelmed. When I asked if there was an acute reason for this, he said that it seemed related to a recent clinical experience that he had had. It involved a patient who was in extreme pain and was dying of cancer. Atlas instructed the nurse to give the patient a certain amount of morphine, to which the nurse objected, because, she said, "We have never given that much before." Atlas insisted that the man be given this amount. A few minutes later, the charge nurse paged Atlas, saying that they were not going to give that amount. Again Atlas instructed them to do so, explaining that his recommendation was within clinical guidelines. The nurse relented and gave the amount instructed by Atlas.

The next day Atlas went to see the patient. The patient, who was crying in pain the previous day, was now able to smile, free from pain. Atlas's prescribed dose worked. But instead of feeling proud (because he was right) and also happy for the patient (who was comfortable), he found himself angry, not understanding why. His anger was not directed at the nurses, though, and he was genuinely confused by it. We went on to talk about other matters.

Toward the end of our conversation, I asked if we could return to the topic of his anger and why he wanted to see me on this particular day. Atlas was eager to do so, for he wanted my interpretation about this experience. I told him that I suspected that this experience with the patient recalled his experience with his brother who died. His feelings were the result of transference. I continued, "My intuition is that you were very upset with the medical team caring for your brother, for mismanaging his pain, and that this anger carried over to this patient. Also, you were angry at this patient because this patient got the care you wanted your brother to have. I think your feelings are actually stronger than anger. I think hate might be more accurate." "These feelings," I continued, "are not rational but they are nevertheless real." I added, "This is not to say that you did not care for this patient as well—you did—but people are often ambivalent about many important matters. Part of you hated this patient, and this greatly disturbed you, which is why you felt you needed to see me today" (cf. the case of Conor in chapter 2).

This interpretation, based on transference, was therapeutic for Atlas because it provided a compelling explanation of his emotional state about which he previously could not understand. It was paternalistic since I claimed to know his emotional state better than he did. Also, my relabeling of Atlas's experience—*hate*—was stronger than his own label—*anger*. This proved to be helpful because, as with the interpretation of the Book of Job, Atlas seems to be searching for more complex understandings of both God and himself. He knows, from his own experience, that God is not simply all-powerful and good. There is a darker side to God. And he is beginning to see this in himself, too. Atlas is not simply a man with the weight of the world on his shoulders. Or, if he is, he is ambivalent about this state of affairs, sometimes fantasying about running away from it all. This relabeling of *anger* as *hate* was therapeutic because it represented, on my part, a fuller acceptance of Atlas.

I embraced him not only in his feelings of anger but also in his feelings of hate; my acceptance of him was even deeper than he had anticipated.

Like Atlas's previous attempts to explain suffering in the Book of Job, understanding anger in himself did not go anywhere. It only confused him. These attempts to understand his own anger may be viewed as attempts at a first-order change. But my relabeling of his anger as hate, based on transference, changed the frame. No amount of reflection on the clinical encounter itself would have freed him from his feelings, for their roots were to be found elsewhere. Like introducing biblical scholarship to Atlas, pointing out the dynamics of transference opened up a whole new world of vision for him, a new frame through which to view his life. This is second-order change. And the fact that his feelings were based on transference also implies that change is possible. Why? Because transference can be worked through.

In sum, I viewed Atlas's life in theological perspective, precisely as Pruyser called for, because this is what he requested. Atlas did not come to me for psychotropic medication or legal counsel—he knew I could not help him in those areas—he came to me looking for theological conversation. Because my perspective was informed by the reframing technique of relabeling, it was inherently paternalistic, but acting beneficently and paternalistically are, as noted, by no means mutually exclusive.[73] I seemed to have done good for him.

A Final Illustration

One of the founding documents of bioethics is Elisabeth Kübler-Ross's *On Death and Dying*.[74] While her five stages of dying (denial, anger, bargaining, depression, and acceptance) are iconic, psychologists today are skeptical of her model, largely because the model does not seem to have empirical support.[75] Nevertheless, health professionals are still taught—and tested on—these stages. While her stages remain extremely influential among medical professionals, it is less widely known that (i) Kübler-Ross was influenced by psychoanalysis in her formulation of this model and (ii) her model is the result of an interprofessional seminar on death and dying in which she took theological students from Chicago Theological Seminary into the hospital to interview dying patients.[76] This was during the 1960s when bioethics had not yet taken hold, and the principle of respect for autonomy was not yet accepted widely. She writes:

> Some physicians favor telling the relatives [that a patient is dying] but keeping the facts from the patient in order to avoid an emotional

> outburst. Some doctors are sensitive to their patient's needs and can quite successfully present the patient with the awareness of a serious illness without taking all hope away. . . . I personally feel that this question should never come up as a real conflict. The question should not be "Should we tell . . . ?" but rather "How do I share this with my patient?"[77]

These reflections from Kübler-Ross might strike many readers as remarkable, because they seem obvious today. Yet, as noted in chapter 2, telling the truth to patients is a recent idea, and it is still to some extent controversial and complicated in some cross-cultural and multigenerational situations. In any case, one can see that the idea of not telling dying patients the truth was grounded in paternalism.

As a final illustration of how reframing techniques might be used in clinical practice, I would like to close with Kübler-Ross's case of Mr. O., a successful and powerful businessman. Mr. O. was hospitalized due to Hodgkin's disease. His wife grew tired of caring for Mr. O. because he became angry and noncompliant. He wouldn't eat when instructed to do so and he gave the hospital staff a difficult time. Exasperated, Mr. O.'s wife came to see Kübler-Ross.

Kübler-Ross explained that Mr. O. needed to feel in control, because this illness made him feel powerless. Mr. O.'s wife still visited him every day in the hospital, but she called him first, asking him when it would be convenient to visit. Kübler-Ross writes: "Also, she stopped giving him advice as to what to eat and how often to get up, but rather rephrased it into statements like, 'I bet only you can decide when to start eating this and that.' He was able to eat again, but only after all staff and relatives stopped telling him what to do."[78] Kübler-Ross continues, "The nursing staff used the same approach by allowing him to control certain times for infusions, changing bed sheets, etc., and—not surprising perhaps—he chose approximately the same times for these procedures as they had been previously done, with no anger or struggles involved."[79] In terms of reframing, this technique is the illusion of alternatives. (Another example of the technique of the illusion of alternatives is when parents ask their children, "Do you want to go to bed at 7:45 or at 8 PM?"[80] This example is, quite literarily, paternalistic, though all uses of reframing techniques are paternalistic to the extent that they are beneficent, albeit less obviously so than the bedtime question.)

While issues such as these (how to get a patient to eat and how to get a child to go to bed) may seem mundane, they really are extremely important, not only to the existential well-being of patients but also to staff. If these problems are not handled with care, they can be made worse, but a beneficent diagnostician with some knowledge of reframing techniques can rescue patients, families, and staff from a living hell. What could be more pastoral than this?

5 JUSTICE AND THE LIVING HUMAN WEB

Imagine while walking down a country road you notice off to the side a small child in need of help because she is in danger of drowning. To save this child, you must act quickly but in doing so you will ruin your shoes, which happen to be your most expensive pair, costing about $200. Are you morally obligated to save this child? This is a thought experiment created by Peter Singer.[1]

Singer argues that one would have to be a moral monster to walk on by and do nothing for the child. It seems that most people would agree. However, Singer further suggests that, while people tend to feel a duty to help a stranger in front of them, physical distance is morally arbitrary. In other words, for a small cost to many people—say, one's most expensive pair of shoes—one can save the lives of several children in so-called developing countries, maybe far away. Yet many people do not feel obligated to help children in distant lands whose lives could be saved with access to clean water and basic medical care.

Singer's thought experiment raises fundamental questions about justice: What is fair? To what extent are we obligated to help others? Such questions regarding the ethics of poverty have been a lifelong interest of Singer. Indeed, he wrote a widely read article provocatively titled "The Singer Solution to World Poverty"[2] as well as a book titled *The Life You Can Save*.[3] Over the years he has tried, with limited success, to get people who are more affluent to give more to others, especially to people who are impoverished in undeveloped and developing nations, because a small amount of money from a wealthy nation can go a lot further there.

Why do people feel obligated to help a child in front of them but not children starving in Africa? Singer suggests that the difference is "psychological" but that these psychological feelings about geographical distance "can make no real difference to our obligations."[4] While it seems obvious that one is obligated to help the drowning child in one's presence, most of us nevertheless spend far more money than we should on material items that we do not need, Singer argues, leading to the preventable deaths of children.

While walking with Singer across the campus of Princeton University in 2002, I asked him how much he gives to charity.[5] He told me that he gives 20 percent of his income to charity. He added, knowing that I was a seminary student, that this is double the Christian tithe. He also stated that he will give a higher percentage when others give more as well. I do not give 20 percent; I admire Singer for doing so.

Singer had a substantial impact on me. I became a vegetarian for about two years because of his views articulated in *Animal Liberation*.[6] While I began eating meat again, I still make an effort to eat meat that has been handled in a humane way. I also give more to charity than I used to but still not enough. I try to do better each year.

Singer, a remarkably clear writer, is a philosopher who thinks universally. Indeed, when I took a class with him at Princeton designed around two of his books—*Practical Ethics*[7] and *Writings on an Ethical Life*[8]—we did many thought experiments in class. One of the most memorable moments from the course was his debate with Harriet McBryde Johnson, a disability rights activist. The focus of the debate regarded Singer's controversial justification of infanticide for certain cases of disability. One scenario in which Singer argued that infanticide is justified is when a child is born with spina bifida. The debate was quite memorable because Johnson was born with spina bifida. After the debate, she published her account of it in the *New York Times*.[9] Love him or hate him, Singer is deeply committed to a particular vision of justice—and he is always unforgettable.

Part One: The Principle

This chapter focuses on justice. In contrast to Singer, I offer a different approach to justice. It is different because it is influenced by several particular strands of critical thought, as will become clear in the following discussion. Also, my approach is focused on an individual. I begin in part one with a discussion of how justice is articulated in *Principles of Biomedical Ethics*.[10] This is followed by two classic cases in bioethics concerning justice: the Seattle Dialysis Committee and the Tuskegee Syphilis Study. They are among the most widely discussed cases in bioethics; both have achieved, as it were, the status of origin stories in the history the field. The former deals primarily with clinical ethics, and the latter with research ethics, and together they illustrate how justice is often understood in bioethics. In part two, I focus on Bonnie Miller-McLemore's pastoral image of the living human web. The essential features of this image include the following claims: (i) human suffering needs to be understood in context; (ii) psychology, while valuable and necessary, cannot by itself make sense of the whole of individual human experience; and (iii) other perspectives and disciplines, therefore, are needed, such as sociology, anthropology, philosophy, economics, and more. In part three I correlate justice and the living human web.

In previous chapters I have used a psychological text or perspective to interpret experiences of illness but in this chapter, following Miller-McLemore, I move to perspectives other than psychology to explore some of the events that occurred at Memorial Hospital in New Orleans, Louisiana, after Hurricane Katrina in 2005. My argument is that a pastoral perspective on justice interrogates systemic sin by attending to local experience, which can affect the weighing, balancing, and specifying of justice. By systemic sin, I mean not personal sins (such as lying) but social evils (such as slavery). In every time and place, both personal sin and social evil are present. In a sense, systemic sin is harder to address because it is not always obvious who is to blame and it is sometimes unclear how to make changes because the problems seem quite large.

Justice

Beauchamp and Childress discuss several theories of justice as well as a number of specific issues and debates, including fair opportunity and unfair discrimination in health care and research, the right to health, the right to health care, global health, resource allocation, and rationing.

Beauchamp and Childress note a distinction between formal and material principles of justice. A formal principle, for example, is that equals must be treated equally. They note that, without providing criteria as to how to determine equality, formal principles such as this remain abstract. An example of a material principle of justice, in contrast, is the principle of need, when needs—such as food and water—are defined. Beauchamp and Childress examine six material theories of justice:

1. to each person according to rules and actions that maximize social utility [utilitarianism];

2. to each person a maximum of liberty and property resulting from the exercise of liberty rights and participation in fair free-market exchanges [libertarianism/neoliberalism];
3. to each person according to principles of fair distribution derived from conceptions of the good developed in moral communities [communitarianism];
4. to each person an equal measure of liberty and equal access to the goods in life that every rational person values [egalitarianism];
5. to each person the means necessary for the exercise of capabilities essential for a flourishing life [capability theory]; and
6. to each person the means necessary for the realization of core dimensions of well-being [well-being theory].[11]

Beauchamp and Childress discuss each of these theories briefly and conclude that, instead of assessing each theory, they will "use them as resources, with special attention given to egalitarian thinking and the distribution of health care and public health resources."[12] They add that they draw especially on the work of John Rawls[13] as well as the influential application and elaboration of Rawls's philosophy by Norman Daniels.[14] Utilitarian thinking also influences their analysis of justice as a core principle in bioethics.

Beauchamp and Childress begin by discussing the rule of fair opportunity. This rule attempts to redress the effects of life's lottery that conveys physical and social health benefits to some and disadvantages to others. They suggest that some in bioethics—such as H. Tristram Engelhardt Jr.—"go too far" when suggesting that disadvantages of various sorts are "unfortunate" but not "unfair."[15] While it may be difficult to determine root causes, many health disparities have been observed along the lines of race, ethnicity, gender, and social status. For example, in part three of this chapter, I discuss the negative health outcomes suffered disproportionately by African Americans after Hurricane Katrina. This was not merely unfortunate; it was profoundly unfair.

Beauchamp and Childress next turn to research ethics, specifically to the issue of vulnerability. They write:

> The notion of a "vulnerable group" was a major category in bioethics and health policy between the 1970s and the 1990s. However, over the years it suffered from overexpansion because so many groups were declared vulnerable—from the infirm elderly, to the undereducated, to [persons] with inadequate resources, to whole countries whose members lack rights or are subject to exploitation.[16]

They focus on economically disadvantaged persons who can be induced to participate in research due to constraining situations (such as lack of food or shelter) and undue incentives (such as perceived large sums of monetary payment[17]). They also note the problem of undue profit, when research subjects receive too little compensation for their efforts.[18] Beauchamp and Childress point out that simply ruling out persons who are economically disadvantaged from participation in research is paternalistic, and, moreover, this deprives such persons of an economic opportunity not otherwise available to them that may in fact be safer than working an accessible labor job in their unique context. It is easy to see how quickly these dilemmas can become complicated, complex, and confusing.

Beauchamp and Childress next address national health care policy, noting that there are two main arguments in support of a right to health care for all: "(i) an argument from collective social protection and (ii) an argument from fair opportunity."[19] Regarding the former, other protections are noted—such as government protections from fire (i.e., fire departments)—and the basic point is that the government ought to provide other similar protections: health professionals can and should protect the public from disease and illness, and this protection should extend to everyone.

Regarding fair opportunity, Beauchamp and Childress write: "Insofar as injuries, diseases, or disabilities create profound disadvantages and reduce agents' capacity to function properly, justice requires that we use societal health care resources to counter these effects and to give persons a fair chance to use their capacities."[20] Yet they realize there needs to be a limit on the allocation of health care resources—spending cannot be limitless—so the terminology to reflect this limit is "a decent minimum."[21] This, Beauchamp and Childress feel, reflects a compromise among the various conceptions of justice previously articulated, though they recognize specifying what this minimum is will be difficult in practice.

Beauchamp and Childress also discuss actions that may lead to the forfeiting of the right to access to health care, such as drinking alcohol. Should taxpayers pay for drinkers who develop liver disease to have a transplant? On the one hand, Beauchamp and Childress note that it is extremely difficult, and perhaps impossible, to isolate single causes of disease, especially given that social forces are also at work in addition to personal habits, so it would not seem fair to exclude persons from treatment. On the other hand, it might be fair for people engaged in unhealthy activities to be required to pay a tax to do so. But would this be, in effect, taxing the poor?

Beauchamp and Childress also discuss statist theories of justice as contrasted with global theories. They note that statist theories focus on justice within the boundaries of a nation-state, whereas global theories transcend national boundaries. The fields of global health and, more recently, global health humanities also grapple with these issues. As intimated by his pond thought experiment, Singer takes a global perspective in his search for what is in the best interests of all, not just, say, the United States.[22] Beauchamp and Childress do as well.

Beauchamp and Childress then move on to discuss resource allocation, the setting of priorities, and rationing. With regard to allocation, they note four types of allocation: (i) "partitioning the comprehensive social budget"; (ii) "allocating within the health budget"; (iii) "allocating within targeted budgets"; and (iv) "allocating scarce treatments for patients."[23] They note that societies need to set priorities to decide how to spend money; there is no way to avoid this. Still, the setting of priorities is often controversial. If a society rations health care resources by age (e.g., by not allowing men over seventy-five access to treatment for prostate cancer), is this ageist?[24]

A recent example of such setting of priorities, Beauchamp and Childress note, is the Oregon health plan. The Oregon Health Services Commission ranked a list of services that established a decent minimum of access to specific health services for all in the state, though this ranking was widely criticized as arbitrary (tooth-capping was ranked more highly than appendectomies) and the list has been adjusted over the years with recurring budget shortfalls.

In summary, Beauchamp and Childress offer, rather than defend, a particular vision of justice, and they apply this vision to bioethics. They describe their vision of justice this way: "We have proposed recognition of global rights to health and enforceable rights to a decent minimum of health care within a framework for allocation that incorporates both utilitarian and egalitarian standards."[25] They note, too, that "no single theory of justice or system of distributing health care is sufficient for constructive reflection on health policy."[26] So, with their principle of justice in bioethics, Beauchamp and Childress strive to assess efficiency, equality, and fairness as they specify justice. Two illustrations from classic cases in bioethics follow to demonstrate what considerations of justice can look like in practice.

An Illustration: The God Squad

In an issue of *Life* magazine, a remarkable article was written by Shana Alexander with the title "They Decide Who Lives, Who Dies: Medical Miracle and Moral Burden of a Small Committee."[27] It appeared on November 9, 1962. Alexander begins by telling the story of John Myers, a thirty-seven-year-old man dying of kidney disease, who lives outside of Seattle, Washington. Twice a week he takes the ferry across Puget Sound to make his way to downtown Seattle where he receives dialysis. At the time this was brand-new technology, and physicians were doing a trial run in Seattle to see if it was plausible to provide dialysis to people in need on a grand scale. This technology—which Alexander called "the first true artificial organ in medical history"[28]—kept Myers alive.

In the 1960s access to dialysis was extremely limited. Alexander writes that each year end-stage kidney disease "kills about 100,000 people in the U.S. alone. Of these 100,000 doomed patients, only one in 50 at present can be considered a suitable candidate" for this technology.[29] At the time, the hospital in Seattle could accommodate five patients, with the cost of $15,000 per patient per year. (Today, the cost is approximately $90,000 per patient per year,[30] and hospitals can treat many more patients.)

A committee to make the decisions as to who should receive this life-saving technology was formed: the Admissions and Policies Committee of the Seattle Artificial Kidney Center at Swedish Hospital. It consisted of seven members: a lawyer, a minister, a banker, a housewife (original term), a state worker, a labor leader, and a surgeon. They became known as the God Squad. While the committee was briefed on medical and social factors relating to each patient, a physician told them that "there were *no* guidelines [regarding ethics], they were on their own."[31] The article contains remarkable quotations from the committee members, demonstrating the many issues that they considered as well as their angst. They had a sense that, even though they were required to make choices, their decisions were arbitrary. They decided, for example, only to consider patients who lived in the state, because their tax dollars went to supporting the hospital. They also considered the commute patients would have to make to receive treatment, their ability to relocate if a commute was not feasible, how many children the patient had (as well as the age of the children), the moral character of the patient (assessed by means of participation in church), whether the patient could be thought to contribute to society after beginning treatment, the patient's will power (i.e., capacity for hope), and the patient's economic status (and ability to provide for one's family after death). The committee also raised questions about the entire enterprise: Do we have the right to make these decisions? Should this money be spent on these patients at all—could more people be helped by directing these resources elsewhere? Where do we draw the line? How should we set limits? It is easy to see how this illustration relates to justice, as these questions all deal with considerations of fairness.

Some fifty years later, Albert Jonsen wrote a commentary in which he noted the God Squad took their work very seriously. Indeed, as one member of this committee recalled, "We always came out of those meetings with empty feelings."[32] As the decades passed, Jonsen observed that the need for this committee and other such committees at local levels became unnecessary, as "policies and procedures," "rules and regulations," and "algorithms and formulas" were developed.[33] He adds: "These are the anonymous, impersonal techniques—a sort of Deistic, not a Theistic, squad—designed to take the agony and inequity out of selection. Technical solutions were formulated for ethical problems."[34] Jonsen does not dismiss the value of this progress, but he does argue that "behind this beneficial and fair field of medical practice looms an ethical problem."[35] It is this: "Behind transplantation medicine is the incessant desire, or rather demand, that life must be salvaged at all costs."[36] He notes that he invokes the word "salvage"—not *save*—intentionally, for it more accurately reflects the battery and wreckage in these attempts to prolong life. This, of course, recalls the principle of nonmaleficence. Jonsen's concern here highlights the fact that more than one principle is relevant to any given moral consideration, as these issues are normally thought of in terms of resource allocation.

There is more in this regard. Toward the conclusion of the essay, Jonsen reflects on his first publication in bioethics, an article that focused on Chad Calland, a cardiologist.[37] When Calland became a patient, he needed a renal transplant, and he subsequently received five kidneys on various occasions, until he committed suicide. On the day of his death, Calland's article, "Iatrogenic Problems in End-Stage Renal Failure,"[38] appeared in the *New England Journal of Medicine*. Jonsen writes: "In that article, Calland complained that his physicians and surgeons had failed to comprehend his feelings about life on dialysis and [his life] after transplantation."[39] Jonsen continues: "He felt he was the object of competition between his nephrologists and his surgeons."[40] After Calland's death, a grand rounds focusing on Calland was held, and his surgeon expressed regret that "in his therapeutic zeal, he had transplanted [Calland] . . . five times with little attention to his desires or feelings, and without sufficient concern for his deteriorating health as one graft after another failed."[41] The use of these two words—desires and feelings—by the surgeon is remarkable, for these words convey both an affirmation of the traditional focus of principlist bioethics (with its emphasis on respect for autonomy) as well as various critiques of principlist bioethics (with their emphasis on experience and emotions). Perhaps Calland's suicide could have been averted had his clinicians practiced a form of bioethics that was more psychologically attuned and therapeutically focused.

An Illustration: The Tuskegee Syphilis Study

Resource allocation (e.g., access to dialysis) is central in discussions of justice. Distributing risk fairly also is central. Indeed, the most influential case in the history of research ethics is the Tuskegee Syphilis Study, a case universally known in bioethics,[42] though rarely mentioned in pastoral theology. The study was conducted by the US Public Health Service in Macon County, Alabama, from 1930 to 1972, and it enrolled 600 African American men (399 men with syphilis, 201 men who did not have the disease), most or all of whom were poor. The case has been widely condemned as unethical for reasons that will be explained, leading to the creation of institutional review boards (IRBs) for scientific research.

Gregory Pence provides some historical context of this case. He notes that social Darwinism—the idea that races are in competition with one another and that inferior races eventually will die out—was compelling to many (white) Americans in the nineteenth and twentieth centuries (and even into the twenty-first as well, unfortunately) and that many physicians embraced social Darwinism. Citing James Jones's *Bad Blood*,[43] Pence writes: "This popular belief [i.e., social Darwinism] was shared by white physicians, who thought that it was confirmed by defects in African Americans' anatomy and therefore [physicians and scientists] became obsessed with the details of such presumed defects."[44] As evidence, Pence offers a quotation from a 1914 article in the *Journal of the American Medical Association*: "The negro springs from a southern race, and as such his sexual appetite is strong; all of his environments stimulate this appetite, and as a general rule his emotional type of religion certainly does not decrease it."[45] In such a racist context, the idea of the Tuskegee Syphilis Study was born.

The experiment was framed as "a study in nature."[46] This meant that the study was to be observational, not therapeutic or interventional. Today, syphilis is treated with antibiotics such as Benzathine penicillin G. But in 1930 little was known about penicillin and it did not become widely available until the mid-1940s. While it is understandable that the participants in the study did not receive penicillin in the 1930s, it becomes less so when these men were not given penicillin as soon as this effective treatment did become widely available. This is one of the most outrageous features of the study. Also, study personnel actively prevented these men from receiving antibiotics into the 1970s.

Prior to the use of antibiotics, the treatments for syphilis involved rubbing metals, such as mercury. In the early twentieth century, a concoction of some six hundred metals, including arsenic, was used, and for a brief time this was thought to be a cure.[47] It wasn't. An irony is that some health professionals at the time suspected that such attempts to cure syphilis with materials such as mercury were misguided and that these rubs were doing more harm than good—so, by enrolling the men in the study, they were *safeguarded* from the standard treatments of the day.

A researcher who believed that arsenic rubs and the like were doing more harm than good was Caesar Boeck, a professor of dermatology at the University of Oslo. With one of his students, J. E. Bruusgaard, he decided to examine the matter further by studying 473 patients who had syphilis by reviewing their hospital charts. Pence writes:

> This method had an obvious bias, since the more severely affected of Boeck's subjects would be most likely to have hospital records. Despite this bias, however, Bruusgaard was surprised to find that in 65 percent of these cases, either the subjects were externally symptom free or there was no mention in their charts of the classic symptoms of syphilis. Of the subjects who had has syphilis for more than 20 years, 73 percent were asymptomatic.[48]

Thus, syphilis was not universally fatal. This provided a significant contrast to the fears of the day. Also, it is important to note that the Oslo Study was of whites. Thus, the rationale for the Tuskegee Syphilis Study, in part, was to do a comparable study in blacks. Yet a major difference was that the Oslo Study was retrospective while the Tuskegee Syphilis Study was prospective.

Perhaps the most egregious ethics violation from today's standards—but also, though to a lesser extent, according to the moral norms of the time—is that the men enrolled in the study were not adequately informed about the nature of the study. Rather, the men were told that they had "bad blood" and that they would receive free treatment and also hot meals for their participation in the study. The men were offered free burials as well, which was attractive to these men because they knew their families would have considerable difficulty paying for a funeral, if they could afford it all. This raises the issue as to whether the African American men recruited for the study were coerced into participating for financial gain.

The study itself was poorly designed and implemented sloppily. While the study was, as noted, supposed to be observational, all of the men in the study received some form of treatment: neoarsphenamine and mercury.[49] The specific treatment given was arbitrary, as this was determined by what was available at the moment. And, because treatment was expensive, none of the men received adequate treatment according to the standards of the day, which, again, was ambiguous. So "untreated" was redefined as "in the modern sense of therapy."[50]

It is not just that the men were not told the whole truth; the men were lied to intentionally. A key physician-researcher in the case explained study enrollment procedures this way:

> My idea in bringing them in large groups is to get the procedure completed in a given area before the negro population has been able to find out just what is going on. Individual patients would be told that they are coming in for an examination but they would remain all night once we had them here, and the details of the puncture techniques should also be kept from them as far as possible.[51]

The "puncture techniques" refer here to spinal taps, which are painful and carry a theoretical risk of paralysis as well (it is not clear that a case of paralysis resulting from a spinal tap has been verified in clinical practice[52]). Later, these men were further misled via formal letters asking them to return for further "free treatment." The letter read: "You will be furnished your meals and a bed, as well [as] the examination and treatment without cost" and concluded in all capitals: "REMEMBER THIS IS YOUR LAST CHANCE FOR SPECIAL FREE TREATMENT."[53] Every aspect of this study provokes moral outrage when the details are examined: lies, racism, and bad science. The effects continue to be felt today, too, for African Americans often mistrust doctors because of this experiment and the wider context of racism in the United States. While IRBs attempt to protect vulnerable populations, they are not capable of restoring public trust. Also, while this case could be viewed through the lenses of other principles—and productively so—in the history of research ethics, this case has been closely linked to justice because it is a clear as well as disturbing example of risks being distributed unfairly in a racist manner.

Part Two: The Image

Having provided an overview of justice as well as two illustrations of it in bioethics, I now want to turn to the living human web to set the stage for offering a pastoral perspective on justice.

The Living Human Web

In "The Living Human Web," Miller-McLemore takes, as her starting point, the pastoral image of the living human document, discussed previously in chapter 2, but in doing so notes a paradigm shift in pastoral theology: "The focus on individual counseling and educative listening has come under increasing criticism from a variety of angles; the prevalence of counseling courses [in seminaries] has waned; 'pastoral theology' has replaced 'pastoral psychology' as the overarching theme; and the notion of care has returned to center stage, with counseling regarded as an important but not comprehensive specialty."[54] Psychology alone, she argues, is no longer sufficient to understand persons and groups, for one must turn to sociology, anthropology, ethics, feminist studies, and more, in pursuing such inquiry adequately. Miller-McLemore pays special attention to the role that feminist insights should play in pastoral theology. She writes:

> A feminist perspective demands an analysis of structures and ideologies that rank people as inferior or superior according to various traits of human nature, whether gender, sexual orientation, color, age, physical ability, and so forth. Hence, to think about pastoral theology and care from this vantage point requires prophetic, transformative challenge to systems of power, authority, and domination that continue to violate, terrorize, and systematically destroy individuals and communities.[55]

So, for Miller-McLemore, the living human *document* is to the individual and psychology as the living human *web* is to social context and multidisciplinarity. To be sure, she argues psychology is still needed; it is just that other perspectives are needed as well.

Miller-McLemore was influenced in part by Catherine Keller's *From a Broken Web: Separatism, Sexism, and Self*,[56] a book that explores misogyny in the west in mythology, religion, psychology, and philosophy. Keller argues that "sexism and separatism—the view of the self as essentially separate from others—are intricately interlinked" throughout western thought and that historically this has led to the devaluing of groups of people, especially women. This devaluing can be observed in various images of and thoughts about women as creatures to be feared (like Medusa) or as objects of desire (like Eve) who are interpreted to have led men astray. Various strands of western thought have functioned to separate men from women, enabling men to be free from the so-called entanglements of women, such as the obligations of family life. Free from family, men can pursue power, status, enlightenment, and the like.[57] Following Keller on this point, Miller-McLemore wants to emphasize alternative myths that stress, in positive ways, the web of interconnectivity. Also, Miller-McLemore notes that the image of the spider spinning a web is poignant because the spider can repair the web, "spinning oneness out of many and weaving the one back into the many."[58] "This mythos," Miller-McLemore continues, "and the theology connected to it have funded a new approach in pastoral theology. More specifically, this means, for example, that public policy issues that determine the health of the human web are as important as issues of individual emotional well-being."[59] (Of note, she wrote an early essay on pastoral theology and bioethics that has inspired my thinking.[60])

So, again, Miller-McLemore is not arguing for the *removal* of psychology from pastoral theological inquiry. Quite the contrary, she argues that women "would do well to retain the power of psychological analysis,"[61] for women need to set the record straight, as it were, with regard to understanding female desire and subjectivity,[62] and they need to speak in their own voice and be heard.[63] Miller-McLemore asserts that each demographic needs to be recognized as contributing to the living human web, showing the depth and complexity of lived experience and realities: "Those within the web who have not yet spoken must speak for themselves."[64] If persons do not speak for themselves and if pastoral theologians do not recognize that some are empowered to speak while other people are not, the potential for misunderstanding the stories of others is great.[65] She concludes: "This lesson—that we must hear the voices of the marginalized from within their own contexts—is one that pastoral theologians have known all along, even when Boisen claimed the validity of his own mental breakdown."[66]

Part Three: Correlation of Principle and Image

While each correlation of principle and image in this book positions materials that draw on psychology, therapeutic literature, experience, and theology, this chapter (because it is informed by the living human web) relativizes the role of psychology and therapy, emphasizing instead other modes of contextual inquiry to explore the case of New Orleans and Hurricane Katrina. Thus, this chapter is an endorsement of the living human web, and as it endorses this image, it focuses on an individual.

A Pastoral Perspective on Justice

For Beauchamp and Childress, justice entails seeking a decent minimum of health care that allocates resources efficiently, equally, and fairly. As a centric force in bioethics, principlist applications of justice tend to focus on, as previously noted, issues relating to health disparities, exploitation in research, access to health care, rationing, and transplantation procedures.

Rather than maintaining this centric perspective, my suggestion in this chapter, in providing an eccentric perspective, is this: *A pastoral perspective on justice requires attention to be given to the local manifestations of systemic sin by listening to the voices of oppressed individuals.* Such a focus can fit hand-in-glove with various liberation and contextual theologies.

When she first articulated the living human web, Miller-McLemore emphasized feminist theological insights, and, as such, the image fits nicely with feminist perspectives in bioethics. An important, recent essay in this regard is Karen Lebacqz's "Philosophy, Theology, and the Claims of Justice."[67] Lebacqz is one of the founders of bioethics who contributed to the Belmont Report, and, in her essay, she makes several arguments that spell out what it means to think theologically about justice in bioethics. Based on her understanding of justice which is derived from the Bible and informed by liberation theology,[68] she argues that a biblically based understanding of justice (i) "implodes" and "explodes" articulations of justice in mainstream bioethics, thereby expanding the scope of justice; (ii) makes central the categories of "oppression" and "liberation" in discussions of justice; and (iii) places the principle of justice "first"—that is to say, questions of justice should have priority over other principles such as respect for autonomy and beneficence. As has been noted earlier, in mainstream bioethics the principle of respect for autonomy often has priority in practice and is sometimes called "the first among equals,"[69] despite the fact that Beauchamp and Childress argue that the four principles are independent and equal. In any case, Lebacqz makes justice primary. The upshot is that the primary difference between Lebacqz's understanding of justice and articulations of justice in mainstream bioethics is that mainstream bioethics, by and large, focuses on abstract questions of distribution and allocation (e.g., Who should receive a kidney transplant?), whereas her understanding of justice focuses on systems of oppression and structures of power (e.g., In what ways does modern medicine exploit people who are poor and other minorities or oppressed groups?[70]). This is what she means by "exploding" articulations of justice in bioethics.

By "imploding" articulations of justice in bioethics, Lebacqz means recovering more traditional understandings of justice by focusing on character formation. These understandings of justice have all but fallen away in mainstream bioethics, although such concerns are making a comeback with various authors writing about professional identity formation.[71]

Placing justice first among the principles refocuses major discussions in bioethics. But what would this look like in practice? An example might be deciding not to build a new neonatal intensive care unit in New York City and instead using the funds and resources on preventive medicine or for nutrition and sanitation in a village in the so-called developing world.[72] The basis for such a decision would not come from abstract reasoning about doing the greatest good for the greatest number but, rather, from listening to the voices of the oppressed. Liberation theology advocates for an "epistemological privilege"[73] of people who are oppressed because all knowledge comes from a point-of-view. Lebacqz, informed by liberation theology, contends that the point-of-view of the oppressed ought to take priority in discussions of justice in bioethics because, as liberation theology suggests, power distorts one's vision.[74]

Lebacqz points out that her conclusions can be reached by other methods and on secular grounds. She cites the work of Iris Marion Young[75] as an example of a secular philosopher reaching similar conclusions, but she points out that theologians were the first to make this kind of a contribution to bioethics and that "the field . . . might yet benefit from attention to categories that are not uniquely theological but have received more emphasis and attention in theological circles than in mainstream philosophical bioethics."[76]

I now want to provide a pastoral perspective on justice by looking at an individual in the living human web to illustrate three strands of systemic sin. The individual is Emmett Everett. He died in 2005 after Hurricane Katrina struck the Gulf Coast of the United States, causing much devastation, especially to New Orleans, Louisiana, where Everett was a patient.

The Case of Emmett Everett

In *Five Days at Memorial: Life and Death in a Storm-Ravaged Hospital*, Sheri Fink provides a journalistic account of the immediate aftermath of

Hurricane Katrina at Memorial Medical Center in New Orleans, based on hundreds of interviews, in which she explored the accusations that a few health professionals hastened the deaths of patients, presumably as an act of mercy.[77] Anna Pou (a physician) and two nurses were brought up on charges of second-degree homicide for the killing of four patients. Allegedly, seventeen patients were killed by health professionals after the storm. Everett was one of these patients. Pou, however, denies these allegations. She also believes that the media has treated her very unfairly. While the following discussion is largely derived from Fink's work, the reader ought not to forget that Pou disputes this account.

Everett, sixty-one-years old, was clinically obese, weighing 380 pounds. He also was African American. At the age of fifty, Everett suffered a stroke that left him paralyzed; he was paraplegic. He was in the hospital before the storm awaiting surgery to help ease his chronic bowel obstruction. He was content with his life despite various health difficulties. When investigators inquired about the death of Everett, it was explained to them that it was felt that Everett was too heavy to carry downstairs to be saved. It has been alleged that there was a discussion about sedating Everett and other patients, so they would not have to wait to die.

A grand jury refused to indict Pou and the nurses who worked with Pou. Pou now refers to her arrest as a "personal tragedy"[78] and claims that she was victimized because of the legal ordeal that she went through. Everett's family, however, feels differently. Fink writes:

> Carrie Everett wanted to see justice done, to see Pou accept responsibility for her actions. Even though her husband, Emmett, had lost the use of his legs and the control of his bladder, and had depended on her care for nine years, she would still rather be bathing him, putting a diaper on him, laughing and clowning and arguing like every couple did—she would still rather have him there.[79]

Since then, Pou has argued for controversial positions in medical ethics regarding disasters and emergencies.[80] She argues that the sickest and most in need of care should be rescued last. This is a reversal of how emergency departments usually operate, where patients in most need of care usually receive it first. Thus, her position focuses on trying to help patients who would benefit the most from rescue (one can imagine Singer agreeing with her). Controversially, she suggests patients with do not resuscitate (DNR) orders should not be rescued in emergency situations. This is controversial because

DNR orders refer to specific clinical situations; they do not refer to evacuation procedures due to a natural disaster. If her position were accepted, it would seem as though fewer patients would agree to a DNR status out of fear of being left behind.[81]

Fink does a good job of raising important issues for bioethics. The issues are sensational: Did Pou murder Everett? When, if ever, are physician-assisted suicide or euthanasia acceptable? When resources are limited during an emergency, who should receive them? Under what circumstances do physicians and other health professionals have a duty to treat during disasters? These abstract moral questions are often debated in bioethics. While they are important to discuss in the abstract, these and other moral issues can receive potentially new consideration by viewing Everett in context of various strands of the living human web.

The Strand of Racism

In *Come Hell or High Water: Hurricane Katrina and the Color of Disaster*, Michael Eric Dyson provides an insightful cultural analysis of Hurricane Katrina as related to race and class.[82] The book is truly interdisciplinary, drawing on history, journalism, public health, critical race theory, and theology.

Dyson begins with a chapter focusing on race and poverty in New Orleans and writes: "When a disaster like Katrina strikes—a *natural* disaster not directly caused by human failure—it frees us to be aware of, and angered by, the catastrophe."[83] He continues: "Even when human hands get involved, our [individual] fingerprints are nowhere to be found [because] we're not responsible for the poor and black being left behind; the local, state, or federal government is at fault."[84] But the problem with this line of reasoning, Dyson points out, is that "we [as individuals] fail to confront our complicity in their long-term suffering."[85]

Was the national response to Hurricane Katrina racist? Because the federal government did not respond in a timely manner to the destruction of Hurricane Katrina (e.g., survivors, including patients trapped in hospitals, remained in New Orleans without adequate aid such as clean water for days), some indeed saw the delay as racist, especially given the media's tendency to describe the behavior of African Americans as "looting" in contrast to whites, when exhibiting the same behavior, who were described as "surviving." What was especially troubling, given the government's delay in responding, was that when the police did arrive they were instructed to stop the "looting" rather than to help the people.[86] If New Orleans were a primarily white city, some argued that the federal response would have been vastly different.

Rapper Kanye West provocatively proclaimed that President George W. Bush "doesn't care about black people."[87] Many were immediately offended by West's remark, including Bush himself, and people who personally knew Bush insisted that he was not at all racist both in this circumstance and in general. However, what Dyson insightfully points out is that West was not referring to Bush's personal attitude but rather to his professional actions. In effect, Dyson was pointing to a distinction between, on the one hand, *personal prejudice*, where an individual does not like a particular group of people (such as African Americans), and, on the other hand, *structural racism*, where a society is organized in such a way that it favors some (such as white people) and disadvantages others (such as persons of color).[88] Dyson adds:

> West was not referring to the president's personal sentiments about black people, which he probably had no way of knowing. . . . West was speaking of George [W.] Bush as the face of government. . . . When West claimed that Bush doesn't care about black people, it was a critical judgement about the failure of government . . . to take care of, in a timely fashion, those citizens under his watch.[89]

Quoting Jacob Weisberg, Dyson writes:

> Had the residents of New Orleans been white Republicans in a state that mattered politically, instead of poor blacks in a city that didn't, Bush's response surely would have been different. Compare what happened when hurricanes Charley and Frances hit Florida in 2004. Though the damage from those storms was negligible in relation to Katrina's, the reaction from the White House was instinctive, rapid, and generous to the point of profligacy. Bush visited hurricane victims four times in six weeks and delivered relief checks personally. . . . The kind of constituency politics that results in a big life-preserver for whites in Florida and a tiny one for blacks in Louisiana may not be racist by design or intent. But the inevitable result is clear racial discrimination.[90]

Theologically, this is an example of systemic sin, as it is not about an individual being prejudiced but rather about government policies that inflict harm. In secular language, this is systemic racism.

In his book, Dyson provides a brief history of the Federal Emergency Management Agency (FEMA) and in so doing details the confusion and hesitation among local, state, and federal persons and groups in responding to Hurricane Katrina. He notes several political gaffes (e.g., after his vacation in Texas, Bush flew over New Orleans rather than landing to visit people). But far more important is the Bush administration's policies, derived from President Ronald Reagan, involving tax cuts and limiting government spending. Why? Because these policies resulted in a disaster much worse than likely would have been the case had the government been attending to civic infrastructure generally and in New Orleans in particular. Indeed, funding to deal with protective infrastructure was cut despite the fact that *these risks were foreseen*. Dyson cites numerous articles warning about the potential disaster of a hurricane hitting New Orleans as well as the likelihood of the levees breaking.[91] Also, Dyson notes that a FEMA report in 2001 emphasized that a hurricane hitting New Orleans was one of the top three threats facing the nation.[92]

In one sense, the key issue concerns limited and diverted resources.[93] The mayor of New Orleans put it this way:

> [The federal government] authorized $8 billion to go to Iraq, lickety-quick. . . . Now you mean to tell me that a place where most of your oil is coming through, a place that is so unique—when you mention New Orleans anywhere around the world, everybody's eyes light up—you mean to tell me that a place where you probably have thousands of people that have died . . . that we can't figure out a way to authorize the resources we need? Come on, man.[94]

But, in addition to limited resources, FEMA also made many confusing decisions and apparent mistakes regarding the resources they did have. Dyson notes, for example, that FEMA turned away aid from various sources (such as Chicago and Germany), mismanaged hundreds of firefighters by not giving them proper instructions (the firefighters played cards to pass the time), and turned away health professionals from other states who volunteered their services.[95]

What does viewing Everett's death in light of the strand of racism do? Viewing Everett's death from this perspective specifies the ways that structural racism contributed to Everett being trapped in the hospital in the first place (due to the lack of governmental spending on preventative maintenance to the levees) and also prevented Everett from being helped in a timely manner (due to the lack of a timely governmental response to the hurricane).

To be sure, neither of these factors suggest that Pou or anyone else was personally prejudiced. The point is, rather, that in terms of justice other geographical areas (such as in Florida) received more attention and resources after less destructive hurricanes—thus, equals are not being treated equally and resources are not being allocated fairly. Viewing Everett's death in light of structural racism haunts us with the feeling that, if Everett were living in a white city, perhaps he would be alive today. More strands of the living human web are relevant.

The Strand of Ableism

In addition to racism, disability likely factored into Everett's death as well. Yet I am not suggesting that Pou or others thought something like, "This man is disabled; he does not deserve to live." Rather, ableism is more subtle. Some basic insights from disability studies can shed light on this form of bias.

In "Disability, Ideology, and Quality of Life," Ron Admunson notes two models of disability: a medical model and a social model.[96] In the medical model of disability, the problems a person with a disability faces in life are seen to derive from the disability itself. If a person is unable to walk, a wheelchair might be suggested. The problem is with the person and a remedy for the individual is suggested. In contrast, in the social model of disability, it is suggested that the problems a person with a disability faces are rooted in social biases against disabled persons. A person who requires a wheelchair to perform daily tasks cannot work in a building if that building is not wheelchair accessible.[97] Thus, the extent to which a workplace or a society takes into account the needs of disabled persons can determine their level of participation. Socioeconomic and political—not medical—factors are key; a person with a given medical diagnosis may be "disabled" in one context but not in another. If in the medical model of disability remedies are individual (and people are helped one at a time), in the social model of disability change is structural (and groups are helped by means of policies, practices, and laws).

Admunson also writes about the common assumption that people with disabilities must have worse lives than people without disabilities. Yet over and over again, an anomaly presents itself when persons with various disabilities are asked about the quality of their lives: "disabled people report a quality only slightly lower than that reported by nondisabled people, and much higher than that projected by nondisabled people."[98] These findings are often reported in happiness studies.[99]

The assumption that persons with disabilities lead unhappy lives is just a step removed from the conclusion that their lives are undesirable, and this sentiment works itself into health care policy and practices in two key ways: quality-of-life (QOL) calculations (cf. chapter 4) and prenatal testing. QOL calculations are often applied to persons with disabilities but the problem with this, Admundson writes, is that "under certain theories of health care rationing, the supposed low QOL of disabled people can imply that they have less claim on health care than nondisabled people do."[100] Pou notes that this was exactly the logic that was implemented after Hurricane Katrina: "The patients were triaged into three groups: A (ambulatory), B (wheelchair), and C (critical). It was intended that the most critical patients would be evacuated first; however, in accordance with triage in a mass-casualty event, the medical staff was told by the rescuers that critically ill patients would be evacuated last, when more help arrived, so that those deemed able to survive could be evacuated quickly."[101]

Relatedly, regarding prenatal testing Adrienne Asch notes that, while she is pro-choice, she is morally opposed to abortion based on prenatal diagnosis.[102] She offers a very critical assessment of bioethics and related fields on this point: "Bioethics, public health, and genetics remain woefully—and scandalously—oblivious, ignorant, or dismissive of any information that challenges the conviction that disability dooms families."[103] Asch argues that health professionals, by assuming that disability is a disaster, actually unnecessarily pressure women into having abortions based on prenatal testing results. Asch, in other words, wants women to have genuine choice.

Asch points out that feminists have argued against selective abortion based on sex because, given the patriarchal and androcentric tendencies of most societies, this would lead (and has led) to the aborting of female fetuses in some countries. Asch also points out that people advocating for what we call today LGBTQ rights likewise would oppose abortion based on our ability to know a fetus's future sexual orientation and/or gender identity or expression, should such technology ever come to exist. The upshot for Asch is that it is curious that some liberal-minded folk think that it is not a bad thing to be a woman or to be gay but that it is, in contrast, unfortunate to be disabled, so much so that it might be better to not have been born. Because mainstream views regarding QOL calculations as well as prenatal testing both reveal an ableist bias, it is not difficult to imagine that ableism played a role in the justifications by Pou and the nurses in allegedly hastening Everett's death.

But what, specifically, did Pou and the nurses do? Writing for the *New England Journal of Medicine*, Susan Okie notes that Pou, in an interview after the grand jury refused to indict her, admitted that "she had administered morphine and midazolam to the ... patients knowing that their deaths might be hastened, but she said she did not intend to kill them."[104] In effect, she invoked the doctrine of double effect as a defense. Okie also quotes Timothy Quill, well-known in bioethics circles for his case of Diane[105] (Quill helped her die), on Pou's administering of these medications: "the drugs Pou gave are typically used for palliation, not euthanasia," and Quill added, "Is it possible they were given an overdose? Yes. But it's also just as possible that they were suffering, that she came through and gave some kind of dose that she thought was appropriate."[106] Thus, Quill does not fault Pou for her actions.

I'd like to point out that theology is often on the forefront of making a case for people who are placed/kept in marginalized groups, as previously noted in the discussion of Lebacqz. Just as feminism in the United States has significant roots in Christianity (the first women's rights convention in the United States was held in 1848 at the Wesleyan Chapel in Seneca Falls, New York), and likewise just as the civil rights movement cannot be understood outside of the context of the Reverend Dr. Martin Luther King Jr.'s religious commitments, disability studies has long had an advocate in theological circles.[107] So, if secular feminists and mainstream bioethicists are unlikely to advocate for Asch's perspective, some theologians (perhaps especially pastoral theologians?) will do so, not from a rigid prolife perspective but rather from a perspective of caring for the least powerful.

The Strand of Anti-Fat Bias

Finally, it is worth speculating about the role that anti-fat bias could have played in Everett's death. My suggestion is that (i) structural racism enabled, by means of various and complex forces, the *situation* that Everett found himself in; (ii) ableism provided a *justification* for the possibility of hastening Everett's death; and (iii) anti-fat bias provoked a *motivation* for doing so. This motivation, masked as compassion or mercy, in fact could have been grounded in an unconscious desire to punish him. If this desire were unconscious, Pou could be completely truthful in maintaining that she did not intend to kill Everett. Pou, seeing Everett lying there fat and seemingly unable to help himself physically, no doubt would have assumed that a doctor—probably many doctors—told him countless times that he needed to lose weight or he would die. Visually, Everett can be seen to have represented in Pou's mind the typical noncompliant patient. In this light, it becomes plausible to imagine that Pou could have considered him to be facing the consequences of not following the doctor's orders.

I realize that such a role for anti-fat bias may seem far-fetched. But, together with the factors of structural racism and ableism (which do not seem far-fetched at all), this suggestion to my mind seems plausible. Indeed, while under normal circumstances (e.g., during a scheduled surgery) it would seem to be inconceivable that anti-fat bias could motivate the hastening of death, post–Katrina New Orleans was not a normal circumstance.

There is no direct evidence that anti-fat bias played a role in hastening Everett's death. But I believe that this bias can be inferred. Like ableism, anti-fat bias is ingrained in health care practices in at least two ways: professional knowledge and personal humor. Regarding the former, in "Prescription for Harm," a chapter in *The Fat Studies Reader*, Pat Lyons offers a historical perspective on today's so-called obesity epidemic. The chapter itself is framed with a striking epigram: "The girth of Americans is increasing. . . . Clothing dealers show that the average American [a decade ago] . . . was easily fitted with a waistband of 46 inches. [Yet today] he requires one of 47 ½ inches. At this rate of increase he will reach [in another decade] a circumference of 49 or 50 inches."[108]

This epigram was taken from *JAMA*. Although it might be thought to be describing contemporary experience in the United States, this quotation was published in 1899—over one hundred years ago! Lyons writes: "Fear of fat is not new, nor is the promotion of pills, potions, surgery, and other 'cures.' What is new in the last fifty years . . . is the extent to which the diet and weight loss industry has moved from the sidelines to the center of American life."[109]

There is today an established body of professional knowledge that pathologizes fatness and also recommends a vast array of treatments for it. Lyons, however, advocates a health at every size perspective. That is to say, she argues that it is possible to be both healthy *and* fat. Being fat does not mean that one is necessarily unhealthy. She adds that, even if being fat were unhealthy, doctors nevertheless should not advocate dieting to combat it, for dieting almost never works: "Of those who enter obesity treatment, most will drop out. Of those who stay in treatment, most will not lose weight. Of those who do lose weight, most will regain it."[110] Again, this quotation is from the *JAMA* article over one hundred years ago but, Lyons notes, it remains accurate even now. Indeed, in the early 1990s one study found that "90–95% of people attempting to lose weight as a part of a weight loss program did not keep the weight off two to five years later."[111] It is possible that genetics account for 70 percent of one's body weight.[112]

Convincing physicians that fatness can be healthy is an uphill battle. Indeed, when a postdoctoral fellow at the McGovern Center for Humanities and Ethics (where I teach) taught a course on anti-fat bias to medical students, few were convinced by the data presented to them—*because this perspective runs counter to their previous education*—though many of them did note that they wanted to study this topic further. In one sense, whether or not fatness is unhealthy is beside the point, because the key issue is that doctors *think* that fatness is unhealthy. Obese patients become coded lazy, noncompliant, and so on, which leads to poorer health care by doctors. Indeed, when patients are obese, doctors often attribute *all* of the problems that a patient might be having to obesity. Gina Kolata notes, in an article for the *New York Times*, that when Patty Nece, a fifty-eight-year-old woman complaining of hip pain, went to her orthopedist, he said: "Let me cut to the chase. You need to lose weight."[113] Kolata adds, "The doctor, she said, never examined her. But he made a diagnosis, 'obesity pain,' and relayed it to her internist. In fact, she later learned, she had progressive scoliosis, a condition not caused by obesity."[114] This is just an example of one way that anti-fat bias can be embedded into the clinical gaze.

Also, behind the backs of patients, doctors and residents routinely make fun of patients, especially obese ones, and this behavior is directly observable and reported often. "I saw the Whale in clinic this week. Her incision looks great!"[115] "Thus spoke a surgeon to a wide-eyed medical student," Michael Kahn writes in an article for the *New York Times*, "who related the comment to her peers (and me) in a group discussion about professional development. The Whale's condition was morbid obesity, and her incision was from weight-loss surgery."[116] The usual justification for such humor, out of earshot of patients, is that it relieves stress, Kahn notes, but in fact such joking is a practice of "othering" patients—that is, dehumanizing them. And if obese patients are "other," it is easy to see why, as was the case for Nece, that hip pain was diagnosed as obesity pain instead of progressive scoliosis.

For all of these reasons, it is not difficult to imagine that during a medical emergency why a fat person might be deemed as not worthy to be saved, especially if they are black and disabled as well. It is too far to suggest that Pou, if she did give Everett an overdose (all accusations are alleged), did so out of intentional malice. Her life as a doctor is dedicated to helping people, as she herself has said. Still, it seems perfectly reasonable to me that unconscious bias could have factored into in her decision-making, especially given the well-established pattern of physician humor about fatness. But, again, it is possible that Fink's account is flawed or biased in some way, as Pou disputes much of the previous discussion.

The Living *Human Web: Experiences of Individuals in Context*

The analysis offered in this chapter represents, in Lebacqz's language, an "explosion" of justice by focusing on structural issues of bias embedded in social and medical thinking, using a case study of an individual's experience. In Miller-McLemore's language such analysis may be understood as an inquiry into the "human *web*" by interrogating issues of racism, ableism, and anti-fat bias. But what about the "*living* human web" or, to use Lebacqz's language, how might an "implosion" of justice be seen to fit with the "*living*" in the living human web? This is precisely where pastoral theology (with its traditional emphasis on psychology, experience, and individuals) is key, as an implosion of justice suggests that the experiences and the views of marginalized individuals ought to be prioritized so that the manifestations of systemic sin at the local level may be exposed and addressed.

The perspective of Andre Gremillion, a nurse who had cared for Everett, is especially helpful in this regard. After the hurricane, Gremillion was agitated by and disagreed with Pou's plans of sedating patients. Fink writes: "He recalled Pou had turned to him in the physical therapy charting room after asking him to medicate Everett and said something like: 'If you don't feel comfortable, don't do it, because it will come back to haunt you. The first time I did it, I wasn't ready and it haunted me for two years.' "[117] Reflecting on this exchange, Gremillion commented, "They were going to give Mr. Everett something to let him go."[118] Diane Robichaux, an administrator, recalled Pou saying, "I know this is hard for y'all, I don't want anybody to feel responsible. . . . I take full responsibility . . . . I don't want anybody to worry about their license."[119]

From a pastoral perspective, what strikes me as interesting and significant is not so much the sensational debates raised by Pou's actions (e.g., Can the doctrine of double effect justify unintentional euthanasia during medical emergencies after disasters?) but rather the personal and moral issues that Gremillion experienced as a disempowered nurse. Approaching Gremillion's experiences in an indirect manner via Fink's account, inferences can be made from literature related to this topic. Specifically, nursing ethics as distinct from medical ethics has developed a large body of literature over the last few decades,[120] and a literature on moral distress, as a kind of subfield or area within nursing ethics, has evolved as well.[121] Two key conclusions from these bodies of literature are directly relevant:

1. Nurses have particular moral insights relevant for clinical ethics that need to be heard.
2. Nurses often suffer from moral distress from not being heard because they are lower on the health professional hierarchy.

These general conclusions can be seen to be relevant to Gremillion's experiences in that he was disempowered by the medical hierarchy to stop Pou from allegedly killing Everett. While he was still conscious, Everett expressed a desire to live, to not be abandoned, but his autonomy apparently was not respected, in the name of justice, according to a controversial ethics of emergencies. My pastoral perspective on justice would give more moral weight to a nurse's perspective—Gremillion's, in this case—and this would have reframed the weighing and balancing of justice.

A complicating factor in this regard is that two other nurses—the nurses who were charged with Pou—seemingly shared a different perspective than Gremillion's. However, Gremillion's perspective as a nurse, together with the wider context of structural racism, ableism, and anti-fat bias, tips the scale in favor of his interpretation of justice. It would have been better to have done nothing—to let Everett die slowly and perhaps even painfully—because his autonomy would have been respected, Gremillion's perspective as a nurse would have been honored, and Everett's family would not have been left with the haunting question: *What if?* If, though, Everett communicated a wish for pain relieving medications, or even a wish to die, Pou's actions could be more readily affirmed. If he did, I would not fault Pou.

Thus, only by looking at the experiences of individuals in context (i.e., the living human web) can moral assessment of a scenario be made with some degree of confidence. Psychology is an especially useful (and necessary) tool for such inquiry, but not the only tool.

A Final Illustration

Each chapter that offers a correlation in this book concludes with a suggestive illustration that I hope inspires further moral inquiry. In this chapter, I have argued that a pastoral perspective on justice requires attention to be given to the local manifestations of systemic sin by listening to the voices of oppressed individuals. This was explored by looking at the case of Everett. But what concerns regarding the present (or the future) might or should we have?

In *Medical Apartheid: The Dark History of Medical Experimentation on Black Americans from Colonial Times to the Present*, Harriet Washington offers, as the title of the book intimates, a disquieting narrative of the many abuses suffered by African Americans at the hands of health professionals.[122] She includes a chapter, of course, on the Tuskegee Syphilis Study, and there are chapters on experimentation on slaves, research on African American prisoners, eugenics and African American reproduction, and contemporary experiments in Africa.

Washington also writes about contemporary research in emergency rooms in the United States. Citing various studies that African Americans historically have presented to the emergency department in greater numbers than whites, and also citing research indicating that these trends have continued into the twenty-first century,[123] she notes that some of these studies are conducted without informed consent when patients are unconscious or not able to consent when they are brought to the hospital.

One of these clinical trials involved an artificial blood substitute, which, if effective, would save countless lives and also perhaps resolve ethical dilemmas for Jehovah's Witnesses who often refuse life-saving blood transfusions for religious reasons.[124] She writes: "Early test results revealed that subjects who received [this blood substitute] instead of blood suffered more adverse events, such as shock, respiratory failure, and pneumonia—and a 49 percent higher death rate."[125]

Nevertheless, many such studies have been approved. And Washington sees racism here: "This disproportionate use of black bodies to perfect cutting-edge medical technology is hardly novel."[126] She adds, "Safe, non-exploitive research into surgical technology is in everyone's best interest, but for African Americans to remain open to such research, medical policies and practices will have to do a better job of shielding black Americans from abuse."[127]

In this chapter I have offered a call for restraint, for it seems better not to act than to regret one's actions later. Regarding emergency room research, surely this work is needed, but before marching ahead in the name of progress, we need to tread lightly, carefully. Yet I do not wish this call for restraint to become a principle or something universal. What I am calling for is something more modest, more personal, more pastoral. What I am calling for is that we bend our ears to the suffering of marginalized individuals before acting, especially before acting on their behalf. Interviews with affected or likely affected persons are needed, just like Fink offered in her award-winning book, as well as old-fashioned conversations, which pastors are skilled at having. How else will we be able to understand the many strands of the living human web? In thinking about what is just for the group, listening to individuals on the margins is not merely useful; it is required. Listening is, or can be, both moral and political.

EPILOGUE

In *Van Gogh's Ear*, a book about the mystery surrounding whether and why Vincent van Gogh allegedly cut off his own ear, Bernadette Murphy notes that Van Gogh's *Ward in the Hospital in Arles* (Figure 6.1), painted in 1889, appears to include Van Gogh himself: "He is in the background reading a newspaper, wearing a straw hat under which there is a band wrapped around his head covering his ears."[1] She continues: "This is a bleak scene: the male patients fully clothed and huddled around the stove for warmth in a vast, echoing room. The staff are stooping and clearly elderly. Next to the stove in the foreground is a coal scuttle."[2] She adds, "There's an unabashed quality to his determination to record events—no matter how troubling, traumatic, or personal—and the painting can be seen as a memento of his struggles."[3] Van Gogh was a psychiatric patient in this hospital.

In the painting there are two nuns; they are not in the center of the action. They are not depicted as engaging patients—their gaze is downcast. Also, there is a cross in the distance at the end of the hall.

Because of the presence of the nuns (who are always a part of a particular religious community) as well as the cross, religion, while not central, plays a significant role in the painting. Also, there is a suggestive use of light in the painting relating to religion. While all of the windows in the painting are open, the area that receives the most light is in front of a closed door. The spot on the floor should be dim, but it is not. This is surely intentional by the artist; it is a means of conveying emphasis, seemingly regarding the cross above the door.[4]

It is not clear who, if anyone, is the subject or storyteller in this painting. Is it Van Gogh himself, sitting and reading? Or is this painting a representation of a perspective from a first-person point-of-view (such as the view of a friend or family member visiting Van Gogh or another patient) looking at the ward? Or is this the view of a doctor or a nurse looking at the ward? Is it the perspective

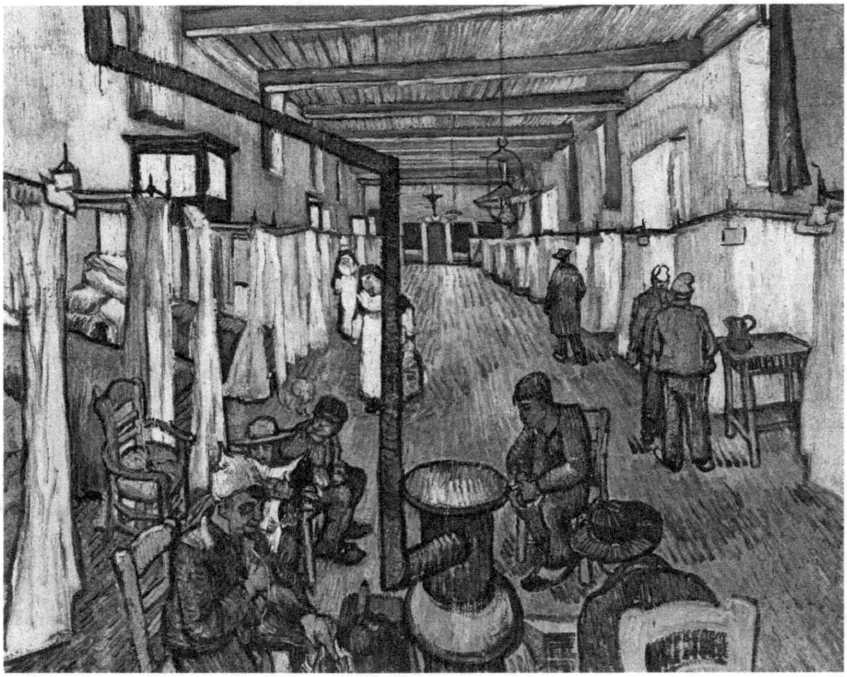

FIGURE 6.1. *Ward in the Hospital in Arles* is a *ca.* 1889 painting by Vincent van Gogh. It is in the Oskar Reinhart Collection, Winterhur, Switzerland. This is a faithful reproduction of a work in the public domain. This work has been identified as being free of known restrictions under copyright law, including all related and neighboring rights: Public Domain Mark 1.0. This work is in the public domain in the United States because it was published (or registered with the US Copyright Office) before January 1, 1923. The source of the photograph is http://www.vggallery.com/painting/by_period/arles.htm.

of another patient? Is this what Van Gogh saw? Is this painting a critique? Is it merely descriptive? Just as the storyteller is ambiguous, so too is the story.

In any case, the center of action involves patients sitting around the coal scuttle, which is, perhaps, an image of hell. The room—both in terms of temperature and in terms of emotions—is cold. Few in the painting seem to be interacting; most are alone together. The long hall could signify the long road to recovery, and, if so, the cross in the distance could be understood to be a sign of faith. Maybe this is, as some have suggested, a clue as to how painting functioned for Van Gogh in general—namely, as a means of conveying despair and cultivating hope.[5]

A Different Approach

Most, if not all, books on religion and bioethics do one of two things: either (i) they offer a particular interpretation of a religious tradition and apply the values from that tradition, so interpreted, to contemporary issues in bioethics (see, e.g., Brent Waters's *This Mortal Flesh: Incarnation and Bioethics*[6]), or (ii) they address epistemological issues, essentially stemming from debates regarding multiculturalism, ultimately making the case that religious voices ought to be included in bioethics (see, e.g., David Guinn's *Handbook of Bioethics and Religion*[7]).

This book has done something a little different. I have advocated for a particular method rather than specific content. My conclusions (which I affirm) are less important than the process itself. Religion in *Ward in the Hospital in Arles*, while significant, is subtle, and I see a similar place for religion in bioethics: significant but subtle. The role of religion in the bioethics that I envision emphasizes *perspectives* more than principles, *aesthetics* more than ethics.

In this book an important distinction has been made between the eccentric and the centric—terms I have taken from art theory. I have associated pastoral theology with the eccentric and principlist bioethics with the centric. The eccentric, as noted in chapter 1, does not mean odd or strange; for me it means both looking *at* and *from* the margins. Over the years I have observed that principlist bioethics, as a centric force, has tended to focus on grand issues (e.g., when does life begin?) while a focus on the eccentric, I suggest, can shift attention to issues that are more mundane (i.e., away from the center) and opens up a wide range of possible inquiry in bioethics. Both the eccentric and the centric are important and valuable.

Based on Van Gogh's painting (Figure 6.1), Table 6.1, organized by principle, contrasts centric and eccentric moral questions. This demonstrates the difference pastoral aesthetics can make.

The centric questions in Table 6.1 each deal with core issues in psychiatric ethics.[8] They deserve to be core. My point, again, is not that centric questions ought to be ignored; my suggestion is that a shift in attention to the eccentric raises different and valuable questions—in this case, in psychiatric ethics.

A Full Harvest

I realize that some with substantial knowledge of pastoral theology and bioethics may feel that this book is old fashioned. Some may feel that another book on *Principles of Biomedical Ethics*[9] is just not needed because bioethics needs to move beyond this paradigm once and for all. While I appreciate such perspectives, I also realize that in academia, because of the requirement to publish to be promoted (and also because publishers have a constant need to sell books), there are market-driven dynamics that reward scholars for

Table 6.1 ***Ward in the Hospital in Arles*****: Centric and Eccentric Questions**

Ethics Principle	Sample Centric Question	Sample Eccentric Question
Respect for Autonomy	To what extent do these patients have capacity?	What is interesting to the man in the straw hat in what he is reading?
Nonmaleficence	Are any treatments (such as bloodletting) harming these patients?	To what extent is religious ideation helpful—or harmful—to these patients?
Beneficence	To what extent is involuntary hospitalization beneficial to these patients?	How can problems in the lives of these patients be reframed so as to free themselves from life-limiting ways of conceiving of themselves or their situations?
Justice	To what extent do these (and other) patients have access to mental health treatment?	What are the social forces that brought each of these individual patients to this place?

pushing into new areas, sometimes prematurely, before paradigms are fully cultivated.

It is my view that insights able to be derived from *Principles of Biomedical Ethics* have not been completely harvested and that pastoral theology has something to offer in this regard—this is why I wrote this book. *Principles of Biomedical Ethics* remains worthy of our *critical* attention. By critical attention, I mean that (i) the principles that Tom Beauchamp and James Childress offered should not be applied in a rote fashion—what Emmanuel Lartey refers to as "applicationism"[10]—and (ii) applicationism can be guarded against via a two-way correlation[11] between principlist bioethics and pastoral theology.

Radiation and Kindness

People are attracted to bioethics because it is exciting and interesting, but principlist bioethics, while helpful, tends to take complexity and context out of classroom discussions. When this happens, Beauchamp and Childress would argue (rightly) that their approach is being misunderstood and misapplied. Nevertheless, my reimagining of principlist bioethics is an attempt to bring imagination back to bioethics, not by focusing on media headlines per se, but by looking for and at the richness of everyday experience. I want health care professionals to listen to their lives. Outside of the classroom, I would like for there to be more venues for conversation.

What I have in mind is something along the lines of the reflexivity found in writings offered by health professionals such as Chris Adrian, a pediatric oncologist who also studied at Harvard Divinity School. "Talking is our procedure," he writes in "The Question," a brief reflection on the question that he always receives at cocktail parties: "How can you do it?"[12] Caring for kids with cancer must be just awful, most people assume. "Sometimes," he adds, "all we have to offer is radiation and kindness."[13] In this deeply moving reflection, Adrian listens to his own life, and in himself he finds that suffering is not denied or minimized, but gratitude nevertheless emerges.

For the last decade, I have attempted to facilitate such listening in the lives of my medical students, and I have found this work to be meaningful and impactful, both to me and to them. I want my students to be kind. I want a bioethics that is kind. And I think that pastoral theology can help because of the discipline's traditional focus on pastoral care and counseling, that is, on listening and talking.

The Central Claims of This Book

The central claims of this book are that pastoral theology can contribute to bioethics and that bioethics can contribute to pastoral theology. Pastoral theology and bioethics, when cross-fertilized, can yield new crops. Specifically, pastoral theology can contribute to bioethics by offering new methods of inquiry and bioethics can contribute to pastoral theology by providing new areas of focus. They offer each other an expansion of territory.

Such cross-fertilization offers a special opportunity for chaplains as practitioners of pastoral theology, for this book serves as an invitation to chaplains to become active contributors to bioethics, not merely passive recipients. This is significant because it has been widely noted that there is a lack of literature for and by chaplains. Indeed, as Stephen Pattison writes, there is "a constant refrain in chaplaincy circles that 'nothing has been written about it' so no one really understands what possibilities and opportunities chaplaincy might offer practically and theoretically, both within and outside religious communities."[14]

I want chaplains, theologians, and others to feel a greater degree of freedom as contributors to bioethics because of this book. I hope that more bioethics materials will be included in theological curricula in the future. Also, I would like for bioethicists to read the work of pastoral theologians.

Pastoral theologians, as noted earlier in this book, have been writing about illness for decades and their work has inherent moral dimensions. Indeed, when bioethicists write about illnesses such as cancer, they would do well to read what pastoral theologians have written about caring for persons suffering from cancer.[15]

A Liberal Protestant Perspective?

Some readers may feel that what I have offered in this book is a liberal Protestant perspective. Such an assessment would be correct, given my own religious heritage. While I offer no apology for my Christian worldview, I would like to add that the perspective offered in this book is less denominational than pastoral. That is to say, more than anything else, my thinking has been shaped less by creeds and confessions than by the thought and writings of Donald Capps (a Lutheran) and Robert Dykstra (a Presbyterian).

The theological perspective on principlist bioethics that I have offered in this book may be summed up as follows:

1. a pastoral perspective on respect for autonomy shifts the focus away from a respect of choice to an appreciation of individuals;
2. a pastoral perspective on nonmaleficence considers harm not only in light of physical and psychosocial considerations but also in light of idolatry;
3. a pastoral perspective on beneficence places an emphasis on existential well-being as influenced by the caregiver; and
4. a pastoral perspective on justice requires attention to be given to the local manifestations of systemic sin by listening to the voices of oppressed individuals.

To be sure, a Roman Catholic or Eastern Orthodox perspective probably would look different than what I have offered in these pages, as would a conservative Protestant perspective. Again, while the perspective offered in this book is particular, what is key for me are not my conclusions but rather this process.

Spirituality and Pluralism

Because of the changing demographics of the global religious landscape, some comments about pluralism as well as the role of spirituality in health care are in order.[16] Regarding the latter, the category of spirituality has gained importance in recent years. This is true in religious studies[17] as well as the health professions. Indeed, for decades there have been movements within the health professions (such as medical humanities[18]) that push clinicians to view patients as persons, not as bodies or diseases. As a part of these movements, treating patients as persons has tended to mean attending to the spirituality of patients.[19]

But what does the term "spirituality" mean? Writing about several different models of the relationship between religion and spirituality, Harold Koenig notes that sometimes spirituality is considered to be a part of religion (as when, for example, Roman Catholic monks are assumed to be more spiritual than laypersons because of their personal devotion), but other times the word spirituality is invoked to be antireligious (as in the phrase, "I'm spiritual, but not religious").[20] Also, spirituality can be understood to include the experiences and expressions of all religions as well as nonreligious persons. Nonreligious persons, for example, might consider themselves spiritual by means of their connection to nature.

In health professional circles, spirituality is understood to be a generic and all-encompassing term. It is intended to be broad and inclusive. Because discussions of spirituality in this context are an outgrowth of patient-centered care, sometimes they attempt to address diversity in health care settings as an aspect of cultural competency.[21] In recent decades many articles have been written on the importance of taking a spiritual history.[22]

This shift to broad and inclusive terms can be observed in other areas. Especially relevant to this book, the term "spiritual care" in pastoral theology competes with the term "pastoral care" because the word "pastoral" has Christian connotations.[23] In health professional ethics, there has been a shift away from the term "medical ethics" to "clinical ethics," so as to be inclusive of nursing ethics and dental ethics. Likewise, there has been a shift from the term "medical humanities" to "health humanities," so as to be inclusive of a wide-range of health professional perspectives on health, illness, and so on.[24] In health professional contexts, it seems likely that the term "spirituality" is here to stay.

What about the changing demographics of the global religious landscape? The Pew Research Center[25] lists projections for 2060. Christianity is expected to increase to 31.8 percent of the world population (from 31.2 percent in 2015), and Islam is expected to increase to 31.1 percent (from 24.1 percent in 2015). Both Hinduism and Buddhism are expected to decline (to 14.5 percent and 4.8 percent, respectively). Judaism is expected to remain the same (0.2 percent). What accounts for Islam's impressive expected growth, especially as compared with Christianity? It is projected that more babies will be born to Muslims than Christians. Another striking statistic involves "nones," that is, persons not affiliated with any religion. In 2015 nones constituted 16 percent of the global population, but in 2060 they are projected to decline to 12.5 percent. Why? This decline is attributed to the fact that atheists and agnostics are aging, and they tend to live in places with declining birth rates, such as Europe, North America, and Japan.

What is the relationship between the pastoral perspectives offered in this book and the fact of multiculturalism? I have several responses. First, I believe that these pastoral perspectives can be appreciated by persons of many different (or no) religious commitments or spiritual persuasions, just like Beauchamp and Childress's principles have been able to be adopted by many different professions, political groups, and countries.

Second, there are many pastoral images; the images and correlations that I have chosen to focus on in this book are just one way of looking at things. I welcome other images and correlations. Indeed, future correlations could be with other pastoral images—Dykstra's book offers nineteen images. One could pursue alternative correlations of the images that I have offered in this book (e.g., the living human web could be correlated with beneficence). Also, there have been more pastoral images presented since Dykstra's book,[26] and surely more will be suggested in the future. That said, I *do* think that the images that I selected are good choices, especially because the living human document is the image associated with the founder of the field, the living human web represents where the field is today, the circus clown is an image derived from hospital chaplaincy, and the diagnostician is an image offered by a health professional (a clinical psychologist). My choices, in other words, are cohesive and coherent.

Third, I also welcome images from other traditions—religious, secular, or otherwise. I can imagine that important images from Hinduism or Buddhism could lead not only to culturally sensitive insights for specific patient and research populations but also to general insights for all patients. What would a correlation of Ganesh and justice yield? Or what would a correlation of Albert Camus's existentialist interpretation of the Greek myth of Sisyphus[27] and beneficence look like? It is fascinating just to ask these questions!

The Letting Loose of Moral Imagination

I concluded the introduction of this book with a discussion of William May on images and moral imagination. I would like to conclude by returning to

May. In "Finding Common Ground in Bioethics?" May notes that "the word 'theory' in its Greek root refers to vision"[28] and that the word "theater" is closely related. He continues: "Theater, like good theory, presents us with a world to see and frees us from the local and the given. Thus applied ethics has a theoretical component related to liberating insight and vision."[29] He continues: "So conceived, moral reflection does not merely scan the world as it is or prepare leaders for the professions as they are. Rather it entails a knowledgeable re-visioning of foundations and ends."[30] He adds: "The humanities open up a wider horizon in which quandaries and systems may be seen for what they are and thus become other than they were. The humanities help correct our perceptions of the world as it appears to the myopia of accepted practice and the astigmatism of vice. To this degree, they help us to serve the worlds in which we work, not perfectly, but better."[31] While acknowledging that this analogy has ableist connotations by associating vision with insight, May's point nevertheless is a good one: the humanities can stimulate our moral imaginations by providing us with wider horizons.

In this book, I have attempted to stimulate moral inquiry by providing a new perspective on *Principles of Biomedical Ethics*. The principles offered by Beauchamp and Childress are not perfect. Principlism has flaws. But pastoral theology (and its many resources) as one expression of the humanities nevertheless opens up wider horizons in which principlist bioethics may be re-understood. Principlist bioethics need not be thin and decontextualized, as it has been so often criticized, for when bioethics principles are correlated with images of pastoral care—a process I have called pastoral aesthetics—moral imaginations can be let loose.[32] Pastoral theology, like theater and like the humanities in general, provides us with tools, including and especially psychology, to liberate us from what we take as given so that we might imagine life in medicine as better than it is today, for patients, caregivers, groups, communities, and societies. Like the unexpected light found by the closed door under the cross in *Ward in the Hospital in Arles*, I have offered a way of looking at things that explores the significant but subtle ways religion can function in the complex lives and complicated contexts of individuals. May principlist bioethics and pastoral theology have a bright and hopeful future together!

NOTES

PREFACE

1. Nathan Carlin, *Religious Mourning: Reversals and Restorations of Psychological Portraits of Religious Leaders* (Eugene, OR: Wipf & Stock, 2014).
2. Paul Tillich, *Dynamics of Faith* (New York: HarperOne, 2009).
3. In addition to the Group for New Directions in Pastoral Theology and the American Society for Bioethics and Humanities, I have presented my ideas at the Cambridge Consortium for Bioethics Education, the Institute for Spirituality and Health (via their blog), and the Program on Religion and Medicine. Articles in which I have developed preliminary ideas for this book include the following: Nathan Carlin, "The Hospital Room as Uncanny: Psychoanalytic Observations and Recommendations for Pastors and Chaplains," *Pastoral Psychology* 58, no. 1 (2009): 27–42; Catherine Flaitz and Nathan Carlin, "Living in Limbo: Ethics and Experience in a Conversation about Persistent Oral Lesions," *Texas Dental Journal* 128, no. 5 (2011): 427–437; Nathan Carlin, "Bioethics and Pastoral Concern: Some Possible New Directions in Pastoral Theology," *Pastoral Psychology* 62, no. 2 (2013): 129–138; Nathan Carlin, "A Psychoanalytic Reading of *A Monster Calls*: Biblical Congruencies and Theological Implications," *Pastoral Psychology* 66, no. 6 (2017): 759–777; and Nathan Carlin, "Medical Religion," in *Religion: Sources, Perspectives, and Methodologies*, ed. Jeffrey Kripal (Farmington Hills, MI: Macmillan Reference USA, 2016), 341–356.
4. This is a line from *Up*, a 2009 film.

INTRODUCTION

1. "Bioethics," *Dictionary.com*, accessed on July 11, 2017, http://www.dictionary.com/browse/bioethics.
2. Stephen Post, ed., *Encyclopedia of Bioethics*, 3rd ed. (New York: Macmillan Reference, 2004), 279.

3. See Jeffrey Spike, Thomas Cole, and Richard Buday, *The Brewsters: An Interactive Adventure in Ethics for the Health Professions*, 2nd ed. (Houston, TX: UTHealth, 2011). Spike organized *The Brewsters* into three sections: professionalism, clinical ethics, and research ethics.
4. See, e.g., Renée Fox and Judith Swazey, *Observing Bioethics* (Oxford: Oxford University Press, 2008), 21–60.
5. Albert Jonsen, *A Short History of Medical Ethics* (Oxford: Oxford University Press, 2000), 116.
6. James Watson and Francis Crick, "Molecular Structure of Nucleic Acids: A Structure for Deoxyribose Nucleic Acid," *Nature* 171, no. 4356 (25 April 1953): 737–738.
7. See Christopher Blagg, "The Early History of Dialysis for Chronic Renal Failure in the United States: A View from Seattle," *American Journal of Kidney Diseases* 49, no. 3 (2007): 482–496.
8. See Johan Brink, "The First Human Heart and Further Advances in Cardiac Transplantation at Groote Schuur Hospital and the University of Cape Town," *Cardiovascular Journal of Africa* 20, no. 1 (2009): 31–35.
9. Ad Hoc Committee, Harvard Medical School, "A Definition of Irreversible Coma: Report of the Ad Hoc Committee of the Harvard Medical School to Examine the Definition of Brain Death," *JAMA* 205, no. 6 (5 August 1968): 337–340.
10. Jean Heller, "Syphilis Victims in U.S. Study Went Untreated for 40 Years," *New York Times*, July 26, 1972, http://www.nytimes.com/1972/07/26/archives/syphilis-victims-in-us-study-went-untreated-for-40-years-syphilis.html.
11. See Robert McFadden, "Karen Ann Quinlan, 31, Dies," *New York Times*, June 12, 1985, http://www.nytimes.com/1985/06/12/nyregion/karen-ann-quinlan-31-dies-focus-of-76-right-to-die-case.html.
12. See Susan Donaldson James, "Test Tube Baby Louise Brown Turns 35," *ABC News*, July 25, 2013, http://abcnews.go.com/Health/test-tube-baby-louise-brown-turns-35-medical/story?id=19764283.
13. See Lainna Fader, "Newsweek Rewind: 30 Years Ago, Scientists Discovered the Cause of AIDS," *Newsweek*, April 24, 2014, http://www.newsweek.com/newsweek-rewind-30-years-ago-scientists-discovered-cause-hiv-248566.
14. Jonsen, *A Short History of Medical Ethics*, 100–114. This long list of events is a paraphrase from Jonsen's history.
15. There is always more than one way to tell a story. See Chimamanda Ngozi Adichie, "The Danger of a Single Story," TED, accessed on December 22, 2017, https://www.ted.com/talks/chimamanda_adichie_the_danger_of_a_single_story/transcript?language=en. On the politics of storytelling in pastoral theology, see Edward Wimberly, *African American Pastoral Care and Counseling: The Politics of Oppression and Empowerment* (Cleveland, OH: Pilgrim, 2006). In bioethics, Tod Chambers writes about the genre of clinical cases as political constructions: Tod Chambers, *The Fiction of Bioethics: Cases as Literary Texts* (New York: Routledge, 1999).

16. Shana Alexander, "They Decide Who Lives, Who Dies," *Life* 53 (1962): 102–125.
17. Fox and Swazey, *Observing Bioethics*, 23–24.
18. Ibid., 23–29.
19. Lisa Cahill, *Theological Bioethics: Participation, Justice, Change* (Washington, DC: Georgetown University Press, 2005).
20. Ibid., 13–42.
21. Albert Jonsen, "A History of Religion and Bioethics," in *Handbook of Bioethics and Religion*, ed. David Guinn (Oxford: Oxford University Press, 2006), 23–35. Regarding the previous discussion, see Nathan Carlin, "Bioethics and Pastoral Concern: Some Possible New Directions in Pastoral Theology," *Pastoral Psychology* 62, no. 2 (2013): 129–138, as well as Nathan Carlin, "The Potential of Pastoral Theology for Bioethics," Institute for Spirituality and Health (blogpost), October 14, 2013, http://ish-tmc.org/potential-pastoral-theology-bioethics/.
22. Daniel Callahan, "Religion and the Secularization of Bioethics," *Hastings Center Report* 20, no. 4 (1990): 2.
23. Ibid.
24. Ibid., 3.
25. Ibid.
26. "The Belmont Report," last modified April 18, 1979, http://www.hhs.gov/ohrp/humansubjects/guidance/belmont.html.
27. The classic book on this history is James Jones, *Bad Blood: The Tuskegee Syphilis Experiment* (New York: Free Press, 1981).
28. Allen Hornblum, *Acres of Skin: Human Experiments at Holmesburg Prison* (New York: Routledge, 1999).
29. "The Belmont Report 25 Years Later—Tom Beauchamp," last modified September 22, 2004, http://videocast.nih.gov/summary.asp?Live=11549&bhcp=1.
30. Tom Beauchamp and James Childress, *Principles of Biomedical Ethics* (New York: Oxford University Press, 1979).
31. Phyllis Beemsterboer, *Ethics and Law in Dental Hygiene*, 2nd ed. (St. Louis, MO: Saunders Elsevier, 2010).
32. See, e.g., Bernard Gert, Charles Culver, and K. Danner Clouser, *Bioethics: A Systematic Approach*, 2nd ed. (New York: Oxford University Press, 2006). Also see Steven Miles's address to the American Society of Bioethics and Humanities after receiving its lifetime achievement award: Steven Miles, "Bioethics and an Ethics of Solidarity," October 20, 2017, http://www.bioethics.net/2017/10/asbh-lifetime-achievement-award-2017-steven-h-miles/.
33. Cathy Graham Nickell, *Uniting Faith, Medicine and Healthcare: A 57-Year History of the Institute for Spirituality and Health at the Texas Medical Center* (La Vergne, TN: Lighting Source, 2012), 33–34.
34. David Guinn, ed., *Handbook of Bioethics and Religion* (Oxford: Oxford University Press, 2006).

35. David Guinn, "Introduction," in *Handbook of Bioethics and Religion*, ed. David Guinn (Oxford: Oxford University Press, 2006), 8; see Michael McConnell, "Equal Treatment and Religious Discrimination," in *Equal Treatment of Religion in a Pluralistic Society*, ed. Stephen Monnsma and J. Christopher Soper (Grand Rapids, MI: Eerdmans, 1998), 33.
36. Cahill, *Theological Bioethics*, 19. Also see Patricia Hill Collins, *Black Feminist Thought: Knowledge, Consciousness, and the Politics of* Empowerment, 2nd ed. (New York: Routledge, 2000); and Diogenes Allen, *Christian Belief in a Postmodern World: The Full Wealth of Conviction* (Louisville, KY: Westminster John Knox, 1989). In bioethics circles, a critique of modern thought has been offered most notably in this book: H. Tristram Engelhardt Jr., *The Foundations of Bioethics*, 2nd ed. (New York: Oxford University Press, 1996).
37. Cahill, *Theological Bioethics*, 19.
38. Ibid.
39. See, e.g., Dariusch Atighetchi, *Islamic Bioethics: Problems and Perspectives* (Dordrecht, The Netherlands: Springer, 2007); and Kerry Bowman and Edwin Hui, "Bioethics for Clinicians: 20. Chinese Bioethics," *CMAJ* 163, no. 11 (2000): 1481–1485. For journals, see *Christian Bioethics* as well as *Health Progress*.
40. Sondra Ely Wheeler, *Stewards of Life: Bioethics and Pastoral Care* (Nashville: Abingdon, 1996).
41. Ibid., 16.
42. If I were to recommend a single book to readers wanting a concise example of theological ethics as related to bioethics, it would be this: James Gustafson, *The Contributions of Theology to Medical Ethics* (Milwaukee, WI: Marquette University Press, 1975). The book is remarkable for its clarity.
43. Gilbert Meilaender, *Bioethics: A Primer for Christians*, 3rd ed. (Grand Rapids, MI: William B. Eerdmans, 2013), 1.
44. Ibid.
45. Ibid.
46. See, e.g., Jennifer Horner, "Morality, Ethics, and Law: Introductory Concepts," *Seminars in Speech and Language* 24, no. 4 (2003): 263–274.
47. Meilaender, *Bioethics*, 3.
48. Ibid., 26.
49. Ibid.
50. Ibid., 30.
51. Ibid., 33. See Mary Anne Warren, "On the Moral and Legal Status of Abortion," *Monist* 57, no. 1 (1973): 43–61.
52. Beverly Harrison with Shirley Cloyes, "Theology and Morality of Procreative Choice," in Beverly Wildung Harrison, *Making the Connections: Essays in Feminist Social Ethics*, ed. Carol Robb (Boston: Beacon, 1985), 117.
53. Ibid., 119.
54. Ibid., 120.

55. See, e.g., Brian Blount, *Cultural Interpretation: Reorienting New Testament Criticism* (Minneapolis: Fortress, 1995).

CHAPTER 1

1. See Erik Erikson, *A Way of Looking at Things: Selected Papers from 1930 to 1980*, ed. Stephen Schlein (New York: W. W. Norton, 1987). I affirm an artistic way of looking at the world, which I have learned from Donald Capps. See especially Donald Capps, *Erik Erikson's Verbal Portraits: Luther, Gandhi, Einstein, Jesus* (Lanham, MD: Rowman & Littlefield, 2014). Also, because of the use of the word "ethical," Capps once directed me to the subtitle of this book: Erik Erikson, *Insight and Responsibility: Lectures on the Ethical Implications of Psychoanalytic Insight* (New York: W. W. Norton, 1964). Through Capps's engagement with Erikson, I have come to appreciate a way of looking at the world that is both aesthetic and moral. Also, Phil Zylla recently has emphasized the role of "perception" in Capps's thought, and Zylla refers to Capps's work as "aesthetic pastoral theology." See Phil Zylla, "Explorations in the Aesthetic Pastoral Theology of Donald E. Capps," *Journal of Religion and Health* 57, no. 2 (2018): 538–550.
2. Robert Dykstra, "Unrepressing the Kingdom: Pastoral Theology as Aesthetic Imagination," *Pastoral Psychology 61*, no. 4 (2012): 391–409. Dykstra's thinking about the importance of thinking about theology as aesthetics is further explored in this book: Robert Dykstra, *Finding Ourselves Lost: Ministry in the Age of Overwhelm* (Eugene, OR: Cascade Books, 2018).
3. Kwame Appiah, *Cosmopolitism: Ethics in a World of Strangers* (New York: W. W. Norton, 2006), 161.
4. See, e.g., Catherine Flaitz and Nathan Carlin, "Living in Limbo: Ethics and Experience in a Conversation about Persistent Oral Lesions," *Texas Dental Journal* 128, no. 5 (2011): 427–437.
5. See, e.g., Jann Aldredge-Clanton, *Counseling People with Cancer* (Louisville, KY: Westminster John Knox, 1998).
6. Tom Beauchamp and James Childress, *Principles of Biomedical Ethics*, 7th ed. (New York: Oxford University Press, 2013).
7. See, e.g., John Evans, "A Sociological Account of the Growth of Principlism," *Hastings Center Report* 30, no. 5 (2000): 31–38.
8. James Childress, "Methods in Bioethics," in *The Oxford Handbook of Bioethics*, ed. Bonnie Steinbock (New York: Oxford University Press, 2009), 17.
9. Tom Beauchamp emphasizes that this framework is neither a moral system nor a theory of ethics. See Tom Beauchamp, "The Philosophical Basis of Psychiatric Ethics," in *Psychiatric Ethics*, 4th ed., ed. Sidney Bloch and Stephen Green (New York: Oxford University Press, 2009), 33.
10. Beauchamp and Childress write "The literature of biomedical ethics virtually never debates the merit or acceptability of these central moral norms, though debates do

occur about their precise meaning, scope, weight, and strength, often in regard to hard moral cases or current practices that merit careful scrutiny." Beauchamp and Childress, *Principles of Biomedical Ethics*, 7th ed., 3.

11. Ibid., 13.
12. Ibid., 17–19. See, too, Tom Beauchamp, "Methods and Principles in Biomedical Ethics," *Journal of Medical Ethics* 29, no. 5 (2003): 269–274.
13. Beauchamp and Childress, *Principles of Biomedical Ethics*, 7th ed., ix.
14. Ibid.
15. See David Ozar and David Sokol, *Dental Ethics at Chairside: Professional Principles and Practical Applications* (Washington, DC: Georgetown University Press, 2002).
16. Richard Miller, "Religion, Ethics, and Clinical Immersion: An Appraisal of Three Pioneers," in *Caring Well: Religion, Narrative, and Health Care Ethics*, ed. David Smith (Louisville, KY: Westminster John Knox, 2000), 17. It is important to note, however, that certain philosophical approaches (such as phenomenological approaches) would not make this mistake, for they do attend to experience in a rigorous way.
17. Ibid.
18. Ibid.
19. Ibid., 18. See Arthur Kleinman, *Writing at the Margin: Discourse Between Anthropology and Medicine* (Berkeley: University of California Press, 1995).
20. In *At the Will of the Body: Reflections on Illness*, a classic pathography, Arthur Frank also makes this argument, emphasizing the "mundane discomforts" that are so central to the experience of being ill. See Arthur Frank, *At the Will of the Body: Reflections on Illness* (Boston: Mariner, 2002), 140. A recent and important book on "everyday ethics" is Larry Churchill, Joseph Fanning, and David Schenck, *What Patients Teach: The Everyday Ethics of Health Care* (New York: Oxford University Press, 2013).
21. William Branch, "The Ethics of Caring and Medical Education," *Academic Medicine* 75, no. 2 (2000): 127.
22. Albert Jonsen, Mark Siegler, and William Winslade, *Clinical Ethics: A Practical Approach to Ethical Decisions in Clinical Medicine* (New York: Macmillan, 1982), 169.
23. Bernard Lo, *Resolving Ethical Dilemmas: A Guide for Clinicians* (Philadelphia: Wolters Kluwer Health/Lippincott Williams & Wilkins, 2009), 3.
24. Tom Beauchamp and James Childress, *Principles of Biomedical Ethics*, 1st ed. (New York: Oxford University Press, 1979), 246–279.
25. See, e.g., Rita Charon, *Narrative Medicine: Honoring the Stories of Illness* (Oxford: Oxford University Press), 2006.
26. John Barbour, "The Bios of Bioethics and the Bios of Autobiography," in *Caring Well: Religion, Narrative, and Health Care Ethics*, ed. David Smith (Louisville, KY: Westminster John Knox, 2000), 43.
27. Ibid.

28. Ibid.
29. Ibid., 49.
30. Anne Hunsaker Hawkins, *Reconstructing Illness: Studies in Pathography* (West Lafayette, IN: Purdue University Press, 1993).
31. Carol Gilligan, *In a Different Voice: Psychological Theory and Women's Development* (Cambridge, MA: Harvard University Press, 1982). See, too, Hilde Lindemann, *An Invitation to Feminist Ethics*, (Boston: McGraw-Hill, 2006), chapter 5.
32. Lawrence Kohlberg, *The Philosophy of Moral Development* (San Francisco: Harper and Row, 1981). Large bodies of literature on both Kohlberg and Gilligan have developed over the decades.
33. See, e.g., Barbara Ehrenreich and Arlie Russell Hochschild, eds., *Global Woman: Nannies, Maids, and Sex Workers in the New Economy* (New York: Henry Holt, 2002).
34. Beauchamp and Childress, *Principles of Biomedical Ethics*, 7th ed., 30–44.
35. Jacob Appel, "Toward a Psychodynamic Approach to Bioethics," *American Journal of Psychoanalysis* 71, no. 1 (2011): 65.
36. Ibid., 59.
37. See, e.g., Joseph Fins, *A Palliative Ethic of Care: Clinical Wisdom at Life's End* (Sudbury, MA: Jones and Bartlett, 2006).
38. Appel, "Toward a Psychodynamic Approach to Bioethics," 61. Appel takes this quotation from Adorno from Donald Moss, "Civilization and Its Discontents: An Ongoing Update. Part 1. The Death Penalty," *Psychoanalytic Review 88* (2001): 87–94.
39. Appel, "Toward a Psychodynamic Approach to Bioethics," 61.
40. Ibid.
41. See Nathan Carlin, "The Hospital Room as Uncanny: Psychoanalytic Observations and Recommendations for Pastors and Chaplains," *Pastoral Psychology* 58, no. 1 (2009): 27–42.
42. Appel, "Toward a Psychodynamic Approach to Bioethics," 65.
43. Thomas Murray, "Psychology Should Be in Dialogue with Bioethics," *Observer* 15, no. 2 (2002), http://www.psychologicalscience.org/index.php/publications/observer/2002/february-02/psychology-should-be-in-dialogue-with-bioethics.html.
44. Olle Sahler and John Carr, *The Behavioral Sciences and Health Care*, 2nd rev. ed. (Cambridge, MA: Hogrefe, 2007).
45. Robert Buckman, *How to Break Bad News: A Guide for Health Care Professionals* (Baltimore: Johns Hopkins University Press, 1992).
46. See Richard Frankel, Timothy Quill, and Susan McDaniel, eds., *The Biopsychosocial Approach: Past, Present, Future* (Rochester, NY: University of Rochester Press, 2003); and George Engel, "The Clinical Application of the Biopsychosocial Model," *American Journal of Psychiatry* 137, no. 5 (1980): 535–544. Jeffrey Spike pointed out to me that many of those who have advocated for the biopsychosocial approach have been influenced by Carl Rogers. It is striking that Rogers also was a

very important thinker for the founding of pastoral theology. While Rogers's influence on pastoral theology has been well documented (see Howard Clinebell, *Basic Types of Pastoral Care and Counseling: Resources for the Ministry of Healing and Growth*, rev. ed. [Nashville: Abingdon, 1984], 42)], his influence on bioethics-related fields is less frequently noted. The term "patient-centered care," which is widely used today (and has been for decades), is borrowed from Roger's term "person-centered therapy" (Carl Rogers, *A Way of Being* [New York: Houghton Mifflin, 1980)]). Thus, there is what might be called a methodological congruence between the historical roots of pastoral theology and contemporary emphases in bioethics that stress narrative and experience.

47. The classic essay on "thickness" is Clifford Geertz, "Thick Description: Toward an Interpretive Theory of Culture," in *Readings in the Philosophy of Social Science*, eds. Michael Martin and Lee McIntyre (Cambridge, MA: MIT Press, 1994), 213–231. Also see Anne Hawkins and Marilyn McEntyre, eds., *Teaching Literature and Medicine* (New York: The Modern Language Association, 2000); and Arthur Kleinman, Veena Das, and Margaret Lock, eds., *Social Suffering* (Berkeley, CA: University of California Press, 1997). The latter volume contains social scientific perspectives beyond anthropology.
48. See Diane Jonte-Pace and William Parsons, eds., *Religion and Psychology: Mapping the Terrain* (London: Routledge, 2001).
49. See Robert Dykstra, ed., *Images of Pastoral Care: Classic Readings* (St. Louis, MO: Chalice, 2005), 1. I have written about the definition of pastoral theology in various places; see Nathan Carlin, "*Middlesex*: A Pastoral Theological Reading," *Pastoral Psychology* 63, no. 5–6 (2014): 561–581.
50. James Dittes, "Some Accidents, Coincidents, and Intents: A Vocational Narrative," *Pastoral Psychology* 52, no. 1–2 (2003): 5–16.
51. Susan Myers-Shirk, *Helping the Good Shepherd: Pastoral Counselors in a Psychotherapeutic Culture, 1925–1975* (Baltimore: Johns Hopkins University Press, 2009).
52. Dykstra, *Images of Pastoral Care*, 9.
53. Ibid. The original quotations in this paragraph are from Valerie DeMarinis, *Critical Caring: A Feminist Model for Pastoral Psychology* (Louisville, KY: Westminster John Knox, 1993), 12–13.
54. Rodney Hunter, ed., *Dictionary of Pastoral Care and Counseling*, exp. ed., ed. Nancy Ramsay (Nashville: Abingdon, 2005).
55. J. R. Burck and Rodney Hunter, "Pastoral Theology, Protestant," in *Dictionary of Pastoral Care and Counseling*, exp. ed., ed. Rodney Hunter (Nashville: Abingdon, 2005), 867–872.
56. Ibid., 867. Emphasis is added here on *from a pastoral perspective*.
57. Ibid.
58. Don Browning, *The Moral Context of Pastoral Care* (Philadelphia: Westminster, 1976).

59. See James Lapsley, *Salvation and Health: The Interlocking Processes of Life* (Philadelphia: Westminster, 1972). Also see Phil Zylla, *Virtue as Consent to Being: A Pastoral-Theological Perspective on Jonathan Edwards's Construct of Virtue* (Eugene, OR: Pickwick Publications, 2011), 104.
60. Burck and Hunter, "Pastoral Theology," 867.
61. See, e.g., this early volume: Peter Homans, ed., *The Dialogue between Theology and Psychology* (Chicago: University of Chicago Press, 1968).
62. See James Woodward and Stephen Pattison, eds., *The Blackwell Reader in Pastoral and Practical Theology* (Malden, MA: Blackwell, 2000). Many of influential scholars of the field are represented in this volume.
63. Dykstra, "Unrepressing the Kingdom."
64. Dykstra, *Images of Pastoral Care*, 2.
65. Ibid.
66. Ibid., 10.
67. Ibid., 12.
68. Ibid., 13.
69. Donald Capps, *The Depleted Self: Sin in a Narcissistic Age* (Minneapolis: Fortress, 1993), 94.
70. Alister McGrath, *Christian Theology: An Introduction*, 3rd ed. (Oxford: Blackwell, 2001), 103.
71. Ibid.
72. Ibid.
73. Paul Tillich, "The Problem of Theological Method: II," *Journal of Religion* 27, no. 1 (1947): 16–26.
74. Ibid., 25.
75. McGrath, *Christian Theology*, 103.
76. Peter Gomes, "Introduction," in Paul Tillich, *The Courage to Be*, 2nd ed. (New Haven, CT: Yale Nota Bene, 2000), xi.
77. Donald Capps, "The Lessons of Art Theory for Pastoral Theology," *Pastoral Psychology* 47, no. 5 (1999): 321–346.
78. See Seward Hiltner, *Preface to Pastoral Theology* (Nashville: Abingdon, 1958); and Rodney Hunter, "A Perspectival Pastoral Theology," in *Turning Points in Pastoral Care: The Legacy of Anton Boisen and Seward Hiltner*, ed. L. Aden and J. Ellens (Grand Rapids, MI: Baker Book House), 53–79. Also see Zylla, "Explorations."
79. Rudolf Arnheim, *New Essays on the Psychology of Art* (Berkeley: University of California Press, 1986); Rudolf Arnheim, *The Power of the Center: A Study of Composition in the Visual Arts*, The New Version (Berkeley: University of California Press, 1988); and Rudolf Arnheim, *The Split and the Structure: Twenty-Eight Essays* (Berkeley: University of California Press, 1996).
80. Capps, "The Lessons of Art Theory for Pastoral Theology," 330.
81. See Nathan Carlin, Thomas Cole, and Henry Strobel, "Guidance from the Humanities for Professional Formation," in *Oxford Textbook of Spirituality*

in Healthcare, eds. Mark Cobb, Christina Puchalski, and Bruce Rumbold (Oxford: Oxford University Press, 2012), 443–450.

82. See Jeffrey Kripal, *The Serpent's Gift: Gnostic Reflections on the Study of Religion* (Chicago: University of Chicago Press, 2007), 29–58.
83. Capps, "The Lessons of Art Theory for Pastoral Theology," 331.
84. See Jane Schaberg, *The Illegitimacy of Jesus: A Feminist Theological Interpretation of the Infancy Narratives* (San Francisco: Harper & Row, 1987).
85. Capps, "The Lessons of Art Theory," 332.
86. Ibid., 333.
87. William May, *The Physician's Covenant: Images of the Healer in Medical Ethics* (Phi ladelphia: Westminster, 1983).
88. Ibid., 13.
89. Ibid., 13–14.
90. Ibid., 15.
91. Ibid., 17.
92. Ibid., 19–20.
93. Ibid., 20.

CHAPTER 2

1. The following is based on a conversation with Jon Wolfshohl on December 18, 2017. These quotations are used with his permission.
2. See Atul Gawande, *Being Mortal: Medicine and What Matters in the End* (New York: Metropolitan Books, 2014).
3. Bernard Lo, *Resolving Ethical Dilemmas: A Guide for Clinicians*, 4th ed. (New York: Wolters Kluwer, 2009), 141.
4. Conversation with Wolfshohl, December 18, 2017.
5. Donald Capps and Nathan Carlin, *Living in Limbo: Life in the Midst of Uncertainty* (Eugene, OR: Cascade Books, 2010), 70–71.
6. Ben Furman and Ahola Tapani, *Solution Talk: Hosting Therapeutic Conversations* (New York: Norton, 1992), 146–147.
7. Ibid.
8. Ibid., 147.
9. Conversation with Wolfshohl, December 18, 2017.
10. Tom Beauchamp and James Childress, *Principles of Biomedical Ethics*, 7th ed. (New York: Oxford University Press, 2013).
11. Ibid., 101.
12. On clinical deception in the late 1970s, see Jerome Groopman, *The Anatomy of Hope: How People Prevail in the Face of Illness* (New York: Random House, 2005), 28–42. Also, a similar point of view was articulated previously in the American Medical Association's 1847 Code of Ethics: "A physician should not be forward to make gloomy prognostications. . . . For, the physician should be the minister of

hope and comfort to the sick; that, by such cordials to the drooping spirit, he may smooth the bed of death, revive expiring life, and counteract the depressing influence of those maladies which often disturb the tranquility of the most resigned, in their last moments. The life of a sick person can be shortened not only by the acts, but also by the words or the manner of a physician. It is, therefore, a sacred duty to guard himself carefully in this respect, and to avoid all things which have a tendency to discourage the patient and to depress his spirit." See Robert Baker, Arthur Caplan, Linda Emanuel, and Stephen Latham, eds., *The American Medical Ethics Revolution: How the AMA's Code of Ethics Has Transformed Physicians' Relationships to Patients, Professionals, and Society* (Baltimore: John Hopkins University Press, 1999), 325. Such deceiving practices, considered for the good of the patient, extend to ancient times, as recorded in the Hippocratic Corpus. See Jay Katz, *The Silent World of Doctor and Patient* (Baltimore: Johns Hopkins University Press, 2002).

13. See, e.g., Leslie Blackhall, Sheila Murphy, Gelya Frank, et al., "Ethnicity and Attitudes toward Patient Autonomy," *Journal of the American Medical Association* 274, no. 10 (1995): 820–825. A recent journalist piece on this topic can be found on the podcast *This American Life*. See Lulu Wang, "What You Don't Know," Act One of Episode 585, "In Defense of Ignorance," *This American Life*, April 22, 2016, http://www.thisamericanlife.org/radio-archives/episode/585/in-defense-of-ignorance?act=1#play.
14. Beauchamp and Childress, *Principles of Biomedical Ethics*, 7th ed., 134.
15. Atul Gawande relays this perspective from a cancer specialist regarding a patient's first visit to talk about prognosis: "I'm thinking, can I get them a pretty good year or two out of this? . . . Those are my expectations. . . . They're thinking ten to twenty years. You hear that time and time again. And I'd be the same way if I were in their shoes." See Gawande, *Being Mortal*, 167.
16. Beauchamp and Childress, *Principles of Biomedical Ethics*, 7th ed., 109.
17. Ibid.
18. Ibid., 111.
19. Ibid., 115.
20. Ibid., 131.
21. Ibid., 140.
22. Gregory Pence, *Classic Cases in Medical Ethics: Accounts of Cases that Have Shaped Medical Ethics, with Philosophical, Legal, and Historical Backgrounds* (Boston: McGraw Hill, 2000). There are many editions and variations of this book. This edition happens to be the one that I own, and I am drawing from it simply to convey key historical facts.
23. Ibid., 31.
24. Ibid., 31–32.
25. Ibid., 37.
26. Robert Dykstra, ed., *Images of Pastoral Care: Classic Readings* (St. Louis, MO: Chalice, 2005), 1.

27. Ibid., 1–2.
28. Ibid., 29.
29. Boisen, quoted in ibid., 9–10. The original text is Anton Boisen, *The Exploration of the Inner World: A Study of Mental Disorder and Religious Experience* (Chicago: Willett, Clark, 1936).
30. Boisen, quoted in Dykstra, *Images of Pastoral Care*, 29.
31. Ibid.
32. Nicholas Wolterstorff, *Lament for a Son* (Grand Rapids, MI: William B. Eerdmans, 1987), 81.
33. James Cone, *The Cross and the Lynching Tree* (Maryknoll, NY: Orbis, 2011).
34. See, e.g., Dan Cohn-Sherbok, ed., *Holocaust Theology: A Reader* (New York: New York University Press, 2002).
35. Patrick Ness, *A Monster Calls*, ill. ed. (Somerville, MA: Candlewick, 2013).
36. In medical humanities, treating the patient as a text has a long history. Ronald Carson notes that, while this metaphor remains promising, "questions about what constitutes the text, and about how the reading gets done, and by whom, continue to be more complicated than we [i.e., medical humanists] originally thought." See Ronald Carson, "The Hyphenated Space: Liminality in the Doctor-Patient Relationship," in *Stories Matter: The Role of Narrative in Medical Ethics*, eds. Rita Charon and Martha Montello (New York: Routledge, 2002), 174–175. Carson credits this insight to Anne Hudson Jones. See Anne Hudson Jones, "Reading Patients—Cautions and Concerns," *Literature and Medicine* 13, no. 2 (1994): 194–195. Alina Bennett directed me to these sources.
37. Carl Elliott, *A Philosophical Disease: Bioethics, Culture, and Identity* (London: Routledge, 1999), xxvi.
38. Rita Charon, *Narrative Medicine: Honoring the Stories of Illness* (New York: Oxford University Press, 2006), 117. Also see Hugh Crawford, "The Politics of Narrative Form," *Literature and Medicine* 11 (1992): 147–162.
39. Elliott, *A Philosophical Disease*, xxiii. Also see Woods Nash, "Showing that Medical Ethics Cases Can Miss the Point: Rewriting Short Stories as Cases," *Literature and Medicine* 36, no. 1 (2018): 190–207.
40. Ness, *A Monster Calls*, 167.
41. Ibid.
42. Ibid., 188.
43. Ibid., 190.
44. Ibid.
45. Ibid.
46. Ibid., 191.
47. Ibid., 203.
48. Ibid., 204.
49. Ibid.
50. Ibid., 205.

51. Nathan Carlin, "A Psychoanalytic Reading of *A Monster Calls*: Biblical Congruencies and Theological Implications," *Pastoral Psychology* 66, no. 6 (2017): 759–777.
52. Sigmund Freud, "On Dreams," in *The Standard Edition of the Complete Psychological Works of Sigmund Freud*, ed. and trans. James Strachey, vol. 5 (London: Vintage, 2001). First published 1901.
53. Sigmund Freud, *The Interpretation of Dreams*, in *The Standard Edition of the Complete Psychological Works of Sigmund Freud*, ed. and trans. James Strachey, vols. 4 and 5 (London: Vintage, 2001). First published 1900. See this text for more recent research on dreams: Kelly Bulkeley, *Big Dreams: The Science of Dreaming and the Origins of Religion* (New York: Oxford University Press, 2016).
54. Freud, "On Dreams," 644.
55. Ibid., 649.
56. Ibid., 651.
57. Ibid., 654; italics in original.
58. Ibid., 655.
59. Ibid., 676–677.
60. Boisen, quoted in Dykstra, *Images of Pastoral Care*, 29.
61. "The Belmont Report," last modified April 18, 1979, http://www.hhs.gov/ohrp/humansubjects/guidance/belmont.html.
62. Donald Capps, *Giving Counsel: A Minister's Guidebook* (St. Louis, MO: Chalice, 2001), 244.
63. Ibid., 245. Capps is quoting Kelly Cannon, *Henry James and Masculinity: The Man at the Margins* (New York: St. Martin's, 1964), 157.
64. Capps, *Giving Counsel*, 246.
65. Margaret Edson, *Wit: A Play* (New York: Faber and Faber, 1999).
66. For a scholarly chapter on the film, see Terrance McConnell, "'She's DNR!' 'She's Research!' Conflicting Role-Related Obligations in *Wit*," in *Bioethics at the Movies*, ed. Sandra Shapshay (Baltimore: Johns Hopkins University Press, 2009), 186–201.
67. For an opposing view (one that argues literature should be used instrumentally for illustrative purposes), see Jeffrey Spike, "How Not to Philosophize with a Hammer: Reply to Montgomery," in *The Variables of Moral Capacity*, eds. D. C. Thomasma and D. N. Weisstub, International Library of Ethics, Law, and the New Medicine, vol. 21 (Dordrecht, The Netherlands: Springer, 2004), 129–135.
68. Donald Capps, *Living Stories: Pastoral Counseling in Congregational Context* (Minneapolis: Fortress, 1998), 59–60.
69. Ibid., 61.

CHAPTER 3

1. Atul Gawande, *Complications: A Surgeon's Notes on an Imperfect Science* (New York: Picador, 2002), 1.
2. Ibid., 1–2.

3. Ibid., 2.
4. Tom Beauchamp and James Childress, *Principles of Biomedical Ethics*, 7th ed. (New York: Oxford University Press, 2013), 150.
5. Steven Miles, *The Hippocratic Oath and the Ethics of Medicine* (New York: Oxford University Press, 2004), 143–144.
6. Beauchamp and Childress, *Principles of Biomedical Ethics*, 7th ed., 153.
7. Ibid., 159–160.
8. Ibid., 162.
9. There is a large body of literature on futility. The most widely cited article on the topic is Lawrence Schneiderman, Nancy Jecker, and Albert Jonsen, "Medical Futility: Its Meaning and Ethical Implications," *Annals of Internal Medicine* 112, no. 12 (1990): 949–954.
10. Beauchamp and Childress, *Principles of Biomedical Ethics*, 7th ed., 178–179.
11. Ibid., 187.
12. Ibid.
13. Ibid., 188.
14. Ibid.
15. Ibid.
16. Thomas Cole, Nathan Carlin, and Ronald Carson, *Medical Humanities: An Introduction* (New York: Cambridge University Press, 2015), 28.
17. Peter Singer, *Practical Ethics*, 3rd ed. (New York: Cambridge University Press, 2011), 125.
18. Ibid., 159–167.
19. Gregory Pence, *Classic Cases in Medical Ethics: Accounts of Cases that Have Shaped Medical Ethics, with Philosophical, Legal, and Historical Backgrounds* (Boston: McGraw Hill, 2000), 176.
20. Ibid., 177.
21. Ibid.
22. Ibid.
23. Marilyn McEntyre, *Patient Poets: Illness from Inside Out* (San Francisco: University of California Medical Humanities Press, 2012), 31.
24. Ibid., 31–32.
25. Ibid., 35.
26. Ibid.
27. See, e.g., this short story by Richard Selzer that explores what it is like for a physician to assist in killing a patient: Richard Selzer, "Mercy," *Iowa Review* 11, no. 2–3 (1980): 117–119.
28. The feminist slogan is: "The personal is political." To say that the personal is theological does indeed encapsulate a major emphasis within pastoral theology from its very inception. An interesting edited volume that also strongly makes this case is this one: Donald Capps and James Dittes, eds., *The Hunger of the Heart: Reflections on the* Confessions *of Augustine*, Society for the Scientific Study of Religion

Monograph Series No. 8 (West Lafayette, IN: Society for the Scientific Study of Religion, 1990); see especially the introduction.

29. Significant volumes in feminist pastoral theology include Jeanne Stevenson Moessner, ed., *Through the Eyes of Women: Insights for Pastoral Care* (Minneapolis: Fortress, 1996); and Zoë Bennett Moore, *Introducing Feminist Perspectives on Pastoral Theology* (New York: Sheffield Academic Press, 2002).
30. Heije Faber, quoted in Robert Dykstra, ed., *Images of Pastoral Care: Classic Readings* (St. Louis, MO: Chalice Press, 2005). The original source in English is Heije Faber, *Pastoral Care in the Modern Hospital*, trans. Hugo de Waal (Philadelphia: Westmin ster, 1971).
31. Faber, quoted in Dykstra, *Images of Pastoral Care*, 86.
32. Ibid., 88.
33. Ibid.
34. This is gender-exclusive language, no longer appropriate for descriptions of ministry.
35. Faber, quoted in Dykstra, *Images of Pastoral Care*, 89.
36. Ibid., 93.
37. Ibid., 92.
38. Jean-Dominique Bauby, *The Diving Bell and the Butterfly* (New York: Vintage Books, 1998).
39. Jason Micheli, *Cancer Is Funny: Keeping Faith in Stage-Serious Chemo* (Minneapolis: Fortress, 2016).
40. Bauby, *The Diving Bell*, 3.
41. Ibid., 5.
42. Ibid., 4.
43. Ibid., 24–25.
44. Ibid., 25.
45. Ibid., 54–55.
46. Ibid., 55.
47. Ibid.
48. Ibid., 132.
49. G. Thomas Couser, *Signifying Bodies: Disability in Contemporary Life Writing* (Ann Arbor: University of Michigan Press, 2009).
50. Ibid., 42.
51. Sigmund Freud, *Jokes and Their Relation to the Unconscious*, in *The Standard Edition of the Complete Psychological Works of Sigmund Freud*, ed. and trans. James Strachey, vol. 8 (London: Vintage, 2001). First published 1905.
52. Sigmund Freud, "On Humor," in *The Standard Edition of the Complete Psychological Works of Sigmund Freud*, ed. and trans. James Strachey, vol. 21 (London: Vintage, 2001). First published 1927.
53. Ibid., 161.
54. Ibid., 162.
55. Ibid., 161.

56. See, e.g., John Morreall, ed., *The Philosophy of Laughter and Humor* (Albany, NY: SUNY Press, 1987); John Morreall, *Comic Relief: A Comprehensive Philosophy of Humor* (Oxford: Wiley-Blackwell, 2009); and John Capps and Donald Capps, *You've Got to Be Kidding! How Jokes Can Help You Think* (Oxford: Wiley-Blackwell, 2009).
57. Freud, "On Humor," 162.
58. Ibid.
59. Ibid., 162–163.
60. Ibid., 164.
61. Ibid.
62. Ibid., 166.
63. Ibid.
64. Micheli, *Cancer Is Funny*, 225.
65. Ibid., 197.
66. Ibid., 200.
67. Ibid., 201.
68. Ibid., 202.
69. Ibid.
70. Ibid.
71. Ibid.
72. Ibid., 204.
73. Glen Gabbard, "Boundary Violations," in *Psychiatric Ethics*, 4th ed., ed. Sidney Bloch and Stephen Green (Oxford: Oxford University Press, 2009), 254.
74. See Charles Taylor, *A Secular Age* (Cambridge, MA: Belknap Press of Harvard University Press, 2007). Also see Larry Shiner, "The Concept of Secularization in Empirical Research," *Journal for the Scientific Study of Religion* 6, no. 2 (1967): 207–220.
75. See Richard Fenn, *Beyond Idols: The Shape of a Secular Society* (Oxford: Oxford University Press, 2001).
76. I have written about secularization and medicine in this chapter: Nathan Carlin, "Medical Religion," in *Religion: Sources, Perspectives, and Methodologies*, ed. Jeffrey Kripal (Farmington Hills, MI: Macmillan Reference USA, 2016), 341–356.
77. Roy Branson, "The Secularization of American Medicine," in *On Moral Medicine: Theological Perspectives in Medical Ethics*, 2nd ed., ed. Stephen Lammers and Allen Verhey (Grand Rapids, MI: William B. Eerdmans, 1998), 13.
78. Ibid., 14.
79. The Mayo Clinic notes: "Smoking causes the majority of lung cancers—both in smokers and in people exposed to secondhand smoke. But lung cancer also occurs in people who never smoked and in those who never had prolonged exposure to secondhand smoke. In these cases, there may be no clear cause of lung cancer." See "Lung Cancer," Mayo Clinic, assessed September 26, 2018, http://www.mayoclinic.org/diseases-conditions/lung-cancer/basics/causes/con-20025531.

80. Branson, "The Secularization of American Medicine," 15–16.
81. Ibid., 15.
82. Ibid., 19.
83. Daniel Callahan, *Taming the Beloved Beast: How Medical Technology Costs Are Destroying Our Health Care System* (Princeton, NJ: Princeton University Press, 2009).
84. Paul Tillich, *Systematic Theology*, vol. 1 (Chicago: University of Chicago Press, 1973), 13.
85. "The Chinese believe that before you can conquer a beast you must first make it beautiful"; see Kay Jamison, *An Unquiet Mind: Memoir of Moods and Madness* (New York: Vintage Books, 1996), 5.
86. Donald Capps, *Laughter Ever After: Ministry of Good Humor* (St. Louis: MO: Chalice, 2008), 107.
87. Ibid.
88. See Robert Dykstra and Nathan Carlin, "At Home in the World: A Memorial Tribute to Donald Capps (1939–2015)," *Pastoral Psychology* 65, no. 5 (2016): 571–586.
89. See Amanda Gardner, "Surgery Mix-Ups Surprisingly Common," Health.com, October 18, 2010, http://www.cnn.com/2010/HEALTH/10/18/health.surgery.mixups.common/.
90. For a recent example, see Danielle Ofri, *What Doctors Feel: How Emotions Affect the Practice of Medicine* (Boston: Beacon, 2013), 39–40. Ofri notes that there are clear rules, even if they are not directly communicated, about how to joke in the hospital, especially regarding the targets of the humor: "Drug abusers are okay; cancer patients are not. Alcoholism and obesity are okay; miscarriage is not. Schizophrenic and borderline patients—yes; terminally ill patients—no. And children with cancer—never." She adds: "Despite sometimes feeling repulsed by the jokes, medical students—and senior doctors too—sense that the humor is not actually mean-spirited, or at least not intended to be. They see the humor as directed at the situation rather than at the patient." She continues: "Physicians of all levels tend to explain black humor in terms of defusing stress and dealing with impossible situations. An ICU physician known for his biting humor once told me, 'Everyone here is dying. What else can you do but joke?'" These casual observations, like many of the other experiences recounted in this chapter, fit with Freud's thesis that humor can help to save precious psychic resources. But it is important to note that it seems as though racial and class biases are built into what Ofri observes as what passes as acceptable humor, for drug abusers, alcoholics, obese patients, and persons with mental illness may be patients who are poor and/or persons of color, more often than rich and/or white patients. Odd as it may sound, dying of cancer may be a form of privilege for persons who have the means to live long enough to die from cancer. Or perhaps the universality of cancer (and miscarriages) carries the fears and anxieties of the rich as well as the poor and therefore is not something to joke about.

CHAPTER 4

1. Daniel Callahan, "Obesity: Chasing an Elusive Epidemic," *Hastings Center Report* 43, no. 1 (2013): 34–40.
2. See, e.g., Christopher Mayes, "The Harm of Bioethics: A Critique of Singer and Callahan on Obesity," *Bioethics* 29, no. 3 (2015): 217–221; as well as A. Janet Tomiyama and Traci Mann, "If Shaming Reduced Obesity, There Would Be No Fat People," *Hastings Center Report* 43, no. 3 (2013): 4–5.
3. There is a small field of philosophical counseling, which often seeks to work with, not against, psychologists (see the National Association of Philosophical Counseling, http://npcassoc.org/), so perhaps it can be in the purview of some philosophers to help people change.
4. Donald Capps, *Living Stories: Pastoral Counseling in Congregational Context* (Minneapolis: Fortress, 1998).
5. Ibid., 70.
6. Ibid.
7. See, e.g., Joan Jacobs Brumberg, *The Body Project: An Intimate History of American Girls* (New York: Vintage, 1998).
8. See, e.g., this clinical article on relational psychoanalysis: Debra Rothschild, "Partners in Treatment: Relational Psychoanalysis and Harm Reduction Therapy," *Journal of Clinical Psychology* 66, no. 2 (2010): 136–149. In pastoral theology, a prominent voice in this regard is Pamela Cooper-White. See Pamela Cooper-White, *Braided Selves: Collected Essays on Multiplicity, God, and Persons* (Eugene, OR: Cascade Books, 2011).
9. This quotation is from this source: Jane Dasher, "Manna in the Desert: Eating Disorders and Pastoral Care," in *Through the Eyes of Women: Insights for Pastoral Care*, ed. Jeanne Stevenson Moessner (Minneapolis: Fortress, 1996), 184. Also see Ellyn Kaschak, *Engendered Lives: A New Psychology of Women's Experience* (New York: Basic Books, 1992).
10. Elizabeth Cady Stanton encouraged women to strive to be regarded as nouns (e.g., "doctor," "lawyer," "professor," etc.), not adjectives (e.g., "hot," "sexy," "thin," etc.) See Jacobs Brumberg, *The Body Project*, ix.
11. See, e.g., Esther Rothblum and Sondra Solovay, eds., *The Fat Studies Reader* (New York: New York University Press, 2009). *This American Life* also produced an episode on this topic: Ira Glass, "Tell Me I'm Fat," *This American Life*, episode 589, June 17, 2016, http://www.thisamericanlife.org/radio-archives/episode/589/tell-me-im-fat/.
12. Tom Beauchamp and James Childress, *Principles of Biomedical Ethics*, 7th ed. (New York: Oxford University Press, 2013), 203.
13. Ibid., 213. They note that they are influenced by David Hume on this point and they provide this citation: David Hume, "Of Suicide," in *Essays Moral, Political, and Literary*, ed. Eugene Miller (Indianapolis, IN: Liberty Classics, 1985), 577–589.

14. An influential essay on this topic is William May, "Code and Covenant or Philanthropy and Contract?" in *On Moral Medicine: Theological Perspectives in Medical Ethics*, 2nd ed., eds. Stephen Lammers and Allen Verhey (Grand Rapids, MI: William B. Eerdmans, 1998), 121–137.
15. Beauchamp and Childress, *Principles of Biomedical Ethics*, 7th ed., 213.
16. Ibid., 204.
17. Ibid.
18. Peter Singer, *The Expanding Circle: Ethics, Evolution, and Moral Progress* (Princeton, NJ: Princeton University Press, 2011).
19. Peter Singer, *Animal Liberation: A New Ethics for Our Treatment of Animals* (New York: Random House, 1975).
20. Singer has made this argument in a number of places. His most rigorous defense of attending to the needs of the global poor appear in Peter Singer, *The Life You Can Save: Acting Now to End World Poverty* (New York: Random House, 2009).
21. Beauchamp and Childress, *Principles of Biomedical Ethics*, 7th ed., 208.
22. Ibid.
23. Ibid., 337.
24. Ibid., 210. Beauchamp and Childress cite a number of articles on breast cancer studies to support this claim, one of which is Rabiya Tuma, "Expanded-Access Programs: Little Heard Views from Industry," *Oncology Times* 30 (10 August 2008): 19, 22–23.
25. Beauchamp and Childress, *Principles of Biomedical Ethics*, 7th ed., 215; italics in original.
26. Carl Elliott, "A New Way to Be Mad," *The Atlantic,* December 2000, http://www.theatlantic.com/magazine/archive/2000/12/a-new-way-to-be-mad/304671/.
27. Beauchamp and Childress, *Principles of Biomedical Ethics*, 7th ed., 227.
28. Ibid., 235.
29. See Nathan Carlin and Donald Capps, *100 Years of Happiness: Insights and Findings from the Experts* (Santa Barbara, CA: Praeger, 2012), 107; and Daniel Nettle, *Happiness: The Science behind Your Smile* (Oxford: Oxford University Press, 2009), 84.
30. Ibid., 239. Also see National Institute for Health and Clinical Excellence (NICE), *Social Value Judgements: Principles for the Development of Nice Guidance*, 2nd ed. London: NICE, 35, https://www.nice.org.uk/media/default/about/what-we-do/research-and-development/social-value-judgements-principles-for-the-development-of-nice-guidance.pdf/.
31. In recent years in the United States a controversy regarding the effects of vaccines has emerged, which is largely anti-intellectual. For a journalistic description of this controversy, see Jef Rouner, "To Protect Other Patients, Some Doctors Are Showing Those Who Refuse to Vaccinate the Door," *Houston Press*, March 17, 2015, http://www.houstonpress.com/news/to-protect-other-patients-some-doctors-are-showing-those-who-refuse-to-vaccinate-the-door-6737198/.

32. Gregory Pence, *Classic Cases in Medical Ethics: Accounts of Cases That Have Shaped Medical Ethics, with Philosophical, Legal, and Historical Backgrounds*, 3rd ed. (Boston: McGraw Hill, 2000), 279–280.
33. Ibid., 281.
34. Ibid., 282.
35. Ibid., 283.
36. Ibid., 285.
37. Ibid., 286.
38. Robert Goodin, "No Smoking: The Ethical Issues," in *Public Health Ethics: Theory, Policy, and Practice*, eds. Ronald Bayer, Lawrence Gostin, Bruce Jennings, and Bonnie Steinbock (Oxford: Oxford University Press, 2007), 117.
39. Ibid., 120.
40. Ibid., 123.
41. Some readers might be interested in the fact that when James McCord, who was president of Princeton Theological Seminary, desired to fill a faculty position in pastoral care, he asked Pruyser if he were interested. Pruyser declined the offer but suggested to McCord that he should hire Capps. The faculty, with the support of McCord, approved the hiring of Capps in 1981.
42. This seems true, at least historically. However, there are many images of and for pastoral care now, as noted throughout this book.
43. Robert Dykstra, ed., *Images of Pastoral Care: Classic Readings* (St. Louis, MO: Chalice, 2005), 161. The original text is Paul Pruyser, *The Minister as Diagnostician: Personal Problems in Pastoral Perspective* (Philadelphia: Westminster, 1976).
44. Ibid., 161.
45. Ibid.
46. Ibid, 169.
47. Ibid.
48. Ibid.
49. Ibid., 166.
50. On the history of pastoral counseling, see E. Brooks Holifield, *A History of Pastoral Care in America: From Salvation to Self-Realization* (Eugene, OR: Wipf and Stock, 1983), as well as Susan Myers-Shirk, *Helping the Good Shepherd: Pastoral Counselors in a Psychotherapeutic Culture, 1925–1975* (Baltimore: Johns Hopkins University Press, 2009).
51. See Richard Fenn and Donald Capps, eds., *On Losing the Soul: Essays in the Social Psychology of Religion* (Albany, NY: SUNY Press, 1995).
52. Donald Capps, "The Minister and Mental Illness," *Pastoral Psychology* 63, no. 1 (2014): 13–22.
53. Personal correspondence, July 28, 2016.
54. Donald Capps, *Reframing: A New Method in Pastoral Care* (Minneapolis: Fortress, 1990).
55. Paul Watzlawick, John Weakland, and Richard Fisch, *Change: Principles of Problem Formation and Problem Resolution* (New York: W. W. Norton, 2011).

56. Ibid., 17.
57. Capps, *Reframing*, 14.
58. Sidney Rosen, ed., *My Voice Will Go with You: The Psychiatric Techniques of Milton H. Erickson* (New York: W. W. Norton, 1973), 149–150.
59. Capps, *Living Stories*, 62.
60. Ibid.
61. Ibid., 63.
62. Ibid.
63. Capps, *Reframing*, 44.
64. Ibid., 44–45.
65. Ibid., 45.
66. I have written about the Book of Job in Nathan Carlin, "The Book of Job and Male Melancholia: A Bizarre Story about Hating Mother God and the Maternal Jesus, Featuring Mel Gibson," *Pastoral Psychology* 56, no. 2 (2007): 121–141.
67. In the Book of Job, Satan is a member of the heavenly court, not God's enemy. See Elaine Pagels, *The Origin of Satan* (New York: Random House, 1995).
68. Capps, *Reframing*, 147–168.
69. See Norman Habel, *The Book of Job: A Commentary* (Philadelphia: Westminster, 1985), 25.
70. Capps, *Reframing*, 151.
71. Of note, Paul Tillich refused to offer an answer to the problem of theodicy.
72. Capps, *Reframing*, 173–177, especially 175.
73. I have been influenced by Atul Gawande on this point: Atul Gawande, "Whose Body Is It, Anyway? What Doctors Should Do When Patients Make Bad Decisions," *New Yorker*, October 4, 1999, 85–91. Also see Kenneth Richman, *Ethics and the Metaphysics of Medicine: Reflections on Health and Beneficence* (Cambridge. MA: MIT Press, 2004), 69.
74. Elisabeth Kübler-Ross, *On Death and Dying* (New York: Scribner, 1997).
75. See, e.g., Michael Shermer, "Five Fallacies of Greif: Debunking Psychological Stages," *Scientific American,* November 1, 2008, https://www.scientificamerican.com/article/five-fallacies-of-grief/. Kübler-Ross first wrote about stages of dying and then stages of grieving.
76. Kübler-Ross, *On Death and Dying*, 35.
77. Ibid., 41.
78. Ibid., 68.
79. Ibid.
80. Capps, *Reframing*, 40.

CHAPTER 5

1. Peter Singer, *Writings on an Ethical Life* (New York: Ecco, 2000), 108. Singer uses this thought experiment in various places and sometimes modifies the wording.

2. Peter Singer, "The Singer Solution to World Poverty," *New York Times Magazine*, September 5, 1999, 60–63.
3. Peter Singer, *The Life You Can Save: Acting Now to End World Poverty* (New York: Random House, 2009).
4. Singer, *Writings on an Ethical Life*, 108.
5. I write about my experience of Singer in Nathan Carlin and Donald Capps, "Consciousness, the Vegetative State, and the Intrinsic Value of Life," *Pastoral Psychology* 57, no. 5-6 (2009): 223–234. Incidentally, this was my first venture into bioethics.
6. Peter Singer, *Animal Liberation: The Definitive Classic of the Animal Movement*, 1st Harper Perennial ed. (New York: Ecco, 2009).
7. Peter Singer, *Practical Ethics*, 3rd ed. (Cambridge, UK: Cambridge University Press, 2011).
8. Singer, *Writings on an Ethical Life*.
9. Harriet McBryde Johnson, "Unspeakable Conversations," *New York Times Magazine*, February 16, 2003, http://www.nytimes.com/2003/02/16/magazine/unspeakable-conversations.html. When Singer moved to Princeton University, protests on campus were organized: Neil MacFarquhar, "Protest Over Princeton's New Ethics Professor," *New York Times*, September 22, 1999, http://www.nytimes.com/1999/09/22/nyregion/protest-over-princeton-s-new-ethics-professor.html.
10. Tom Beauchamp and James Childress, *Principles of Biomedical Ethics*, 7th ed. (New York: Oxford University Press, 2013).
11. Ibid., 253.
12. Ibid., 262.
13. See John Rawls, *A Theory of Justice*, rev. ed. (Cambridge, MA: Belknap Press of Harvard University Press, 1999).
14. See Norman Daniels, *Just Health Care: Studies in Philosophy and Health Policy* (Cambridge, UK: Cambridge University Press, 1985).
15. Beauchamp and Childress, *Principles of Biomedical Ethics*, 7th ed., 264; See H. Tristram Engelhardt Jr., *The Foundations of Bioethics*, 2nd ed. (New York: Oxford University Press, 1996), 382–384.
16. Beauchamp and Childress, *Principles of Biomedical Ethics*, 7th ed., 267.
17. Carl Elliott, *White Coat, Black Hat: Adventures on the Dark Side of Medicine* (Boston: Beacon, 2010), 146.
18. Ibid., 1-23.
19. Beauchamp and Childress, *Principles of Biomedical Ethics*, 7th ed., 271.
20. Ibid., 272.
21. Ibid.
22. See Peter Singer, *One World: The Ethics of Globalization* (New Haven, CT: Yale University Press, 2002).
23. Beauchamp and Childress, *Principles of Biomedical Ethics*, 7th ed., 279–280.

24. See Daniel Callahan, *Setting Limits: Medical Goals in an Aging Society* (New York: Simon and Schuster, 1987).
25. Beauchamp and Childress, *Principles of Biomedical Ethics*, 7th ed., 293.
26. Ibid., 292–293.
27. Shana Alexander, "They Decide Who Lives, Who Dies: Medical Miracle and Moral Burden of a Small Committee," *Life*, November 9, 1962, 102–125.
28. Ibid., 103.
29. Ibid., 104.
30. The University of California, San Francisco, "The Kidney Project," August 7, 2017, https://pharm.ucsf.edu/kidney/need/statistics.
31. Alexander, "They Decide Who Lives, Who Dies," 106.
32. Albert Jonsen, "The God Squad and the Origins of Transplantation Ethics and Policy," *Journal of Law, Medicine and Ethics* 35, no. 2 (2007): 238.
33. Ibid., 239.
34. Ibid.
35. Ibid.
36. Ibid.
37. Albert Jonsen, "Scientific Medicine and Therapeutic Choice," *New England Journal of Medicine*, 292 (1975): 126–127.
38. Chad Calland, "Iatrogenic Problems in End-Stage Renal Failure," *New England Journal of Medicine* 287 (1972): 334–336.
39. Jonsen, "Scientific Medicine and Therapeutic Choice," 240.
40. Ibid.
41. Ibid.
42. See, e.g., Allan Brandt, "Racism and Research: The Case of the Tuskegee Syphilis Study," in *Ethical and Regulatory Aspects of Clinical Research: Readings and Commentary*, ed. Ezekiel Emanuel, Robert Crouch, John Arras, Jonathan Moreno, and Christie Grady (Baltimore: Johns Hopkins University Press, 2003), 20–23.
43. James Jones, *Bad Blood: The Tuskegee Syphilis Experiment*, new exp. ed. (New York: Free Press, 1993).
44. Gregory Pence, *Classic Cases in Medical Ethics: Accounts of Cases that Have Shaped Medical Ethics, with Philosophical, Legal, and Historical Backgrounds*, 3rd ed. (Boston: McGraw Hill, 2000), 256.
45. Ibid.
46. Ibid., 257.
47. Ibid., 255.
48. Ibid.
49. Jones, *Bad Blood*, 119.
50. Ibid., 126.
51. Ibid., 123.
52. Jon Wolfshohl, an emergency medicine physician, informed me of this common misconception or assumption.

53. Jones, *Bad Blood*, 127.
54. Bonnie Miller-McLemore, quoted in Robert Dykstra, ed., *Images of Pastoral Care: Classic Readings* (St. Louis, MO: Chalice, 2005), 40. The original publication is Bonnie Miller-McLemore, "The Human Web: Reflections on the State of Pastoral Theology," *Christian Century* (1993): 366–369. This article was expanded into a book chapter: Bonnie Miller-McLemore, "The Living Human Web: Pastoral Theology at the Turn of the Century," in *Through the Eyes of Women: Insights for Pastoral Care*, ed. Jeanne Stevenson Moessner (Minneapolis: Fortress, 1996), 9–26. She continued to develop her ideas in Bonnie Miller-McLemore, "Revisiting the Living Human Web: Theological Education and the Role of Clinical Pastoral Education," *Journal of Pastoral Care and Counseling* 62, no. 1-2 (2008): 3–18; and Bonnie Miller-McLemore, "Pastoral Theology as Public Theology: Revolutions in the 'Fourth Area,'" ed. Nancy Ramsay, *Pastoral Care and Counseling: Redefining the Paradigms* (Nashville: Abingdon, 2004), 44–64. Her most recent essay is Bonnie Miller-McLemore, "The Living Human Web: A Twenty-Five Year Retrospective," *Pastoral Psychology* 67, no. 3 (2018): 305–321. In speaking with Miller-McLemore about the image, the key development over the years, for her, is seeing the living human document *in* in the living human web. In other words, rather than emphasizing the differences between the living human document and the living human web, she now prefers to combine the images and to see them together.
55. Miller-McLemore, quoted in Dykstra, *Images*, 41.
56. Catherine Keller, *From a Broken Web: Separation, Sexism, and Self* (Boston: Beacon, 1986).
57. Such sexist assessments of family life from men's perspective, of course, are not limited to western culture. The Hindu mystic Ramakrishna was sharply critical of family life, referring to mother and children as "the bitch and the kids." See Jeffrey Kripal, *Kali's Child: The Mystical and the Erotic in the Life and Teachings of Ramakrishna* (Chicago: University of Chicago Press, 1995), 281.
58. Miller-McLemore, quoted in Dykstra, *Images of Pastoral Care*, 42.
59. Ibid., 42–43.
60. Bonnie Miller-McLemore, "Thinking Theologically about Modern Medicine," *Journal of Religion and Health* 30, no. 4 (1991): 287–298.
61. Miller-McLemore, quoted in Dykstra, *Images of Pastoral Care*, 43.
62. See Juliet Mitchell, *Psychoanalysis and Feminism* (New York: Basic Books, 2000); also see Pamela Cooper-White, *Many Voices: Pastoral Psychotherapy in Relational and Theological Perspective* (Minneapolis: Fortress, 2007).
63. An important essay in feminist criticism needs to be noted: Patti Lather, "Postbook: Working the Ruins of Feminist Ethnography," *Signs* 27, no. 1 (2001): 199–227.
64. Miller-McLemore, quoted in Dykstra, *Images of Pastoral Care*, 46.
65. See Melinda McGarrah Sharp, *Misunderstanding Stories: Toward a Postcolonial Pastoral Theology* (Eugene, OR: Pickwick Publications, 2013).

66. Miller-McLemore, quoted in Dykstra, *Images of Pastoral Care*, 46.
67. Karen Lebacqz, "Philosophy, Theology, and the Claims of Justice," in *Handbook of Bioethics and Religion*, ed David Guinn (Oxford: Oxford University Press, 2006), 253–263. This discussion appears in a previous article that I have published: Nathan Carlin, "Bioethics and Pastoral Concern: Some Possible New Directions in Pastoral Theology," *Pastoral Psychology* 62, no. 2 (2013): 129–138.
68. Gustavo Gutiérrez is often considered the founder of liberation theology. See Gustavo Gutiérrez, *A Theology of Liberation: History Politics, and Salvation*, rev. ed., trans. and ed. Caridad Inda and John Eagleson (Maryknoll, NY: Orbis, 1988). Rubem Alves also may be considered a founder of liberation theology.
69. Raanan Gillon, "Ethics Needs Principles—Four Can Encompass the Rest—and Respect for Autonomy Should Be "First among Equals," *Journal of Medical Ethics* 29 (2003): 307–312.
70. See, e.g., Jonathan Metzl, *The Protest Psychosis: How Schizophrenia became a Black Disease* (Boston: Beacon, 2009). Also, Metzl is associated with "structural competency" in medical education: Jonathan Metzl and Helena Hansen, "Structural Competency: Theorizing a New Medical Engagement with Stigma and Inequality," *Social Science and Medicine* 103 (2014): 126–133.
71. Thomas Inui, *A Flag in the Wind: Educating for Professionalism in Medicine* (Washington, DC: Association of American Medical Colleges, 2003).
72. Helga Kuhse and Peter Singer, eds., *A Companion to Bioethics*, 2nd ed. (Malden, MA: Wiley-Blackwell, 2009), 10–11.
73. While I first learned of the term "epistemological privilege" from Brian Blount and Mark Taylor, a recent essay demonstrating its usage is Melissa Browning, "Epistemological Privilege and Collaborative Research: A Reflection on Researching as an Outsider," *Practical Matters* 6 (2013): 1–16.
74. Gutiérrez, *A Theology of Liberation*; Norbert Lohfink, *Option for the Poor: The Basic Principle of Liberation Theology in Light of the Bible*, 2nd ed., trans. Linda Maloney, ed. Duane Christensen (North Richland Hills, TX: Bibal, 1995).
75. Iris Marion Young, *Justice and the Politics of Difference* (Princeton, NJ: Princeton University Press, 1990).
76. Lebacqz, "Philosophy, Theology, and the Claims of Justice," 260.
77. Sheri Fink, *Five Days at Memorial: Life and Death in a Storm-Ravaged Hospital* (New York: Broadway Books, 2013).
78. Sheri Fink, "The Deadly Choices at Memorial," *New York Times*, August 25, 2009, http://www.nytimes.com/2009/08/30/magazine/30doctors.html?pagewanted=all.
79. Fink, *Five Days at Memorial*, 444.
80. Fink, "The Deadly Choices at Memorial." Fink notes that Pou "argues for changing the standards of medical care in emergencies. She has said that informed consent is impossible during disasters and that doctors need to be able to evacuate the sickest or most severely injured patients last—along with those who have

Do Not Resuscitate orders—an approach that she and her colleagues used as conditions worsened after Katrina."

81. See Amanda Schaffer, "The Moral Dilemmas of Doctors During Disasters," *New Yorker,* September 12, 2013, https://www.newyorker.com/tech/elements/the-moral-dilemmas-of-doctors-during-disaster.
82. Michael Eric Dyson, *Come Hell or High Water: Hurricane Katrina and the Color of Disaster* (New York: Basic Civitas, 2005).
83. Ibid., 3.
84. Ibid., 4.
85. Ibid.
86. Ibid., 164.
87. Ibid., 27.
88. See Joe Feagin and Zinobia Bennefield, "Systemic Racism and U.S. Health Care," *Social Science and Medicine* 103 (2014): 7–14.
89. Dyson, *Come Hell or High Water*, 28–29.
90. Ibid., 31.
91. Ibid., 70.
92. Ibid., 78.
93. Ibid., 113.
94. Ibid., 93.
95. Ibid., 124–125.
96. Ron Admunson, "Disability, Ideology, and Quality of Life: A Bias in Biomedical Ethics," in *Quality of Life and Human Difference: Genetic Testing, Health Care, and Disability*, eds. David Wasserman, Jerome Bickenbach, and Robert Wachbroit (Cambridge, UK: Cambridge University Press, 2005), 101–124.
97. In pastoral theology Phil Zylla is a poignant voice on disability and church life: Phil Zylla, "Practices of Acceptance, Understanding and Reciprocity: Caring for Children with Disabilities and their Families," *Pastoral Psychology* 65, no. 5 (2016): 703–715. Out of protest and solidarity, Zylla will not enter a building if it is not wheelchair accessible.
98. Admunson, "Disability, Ideology, and Quality of Life," 103.
99. For a discussion on the problem of subjectivity and assessing another person's happiness, see Nathan Carlin and Donald Capps, *100 Years of Happiness: Insights and Findings from the Experts* (Santa Barbara, CA: Praeger, 2012), 116–118; also see Martin Seligman, *Authentic Happiness: Using the New Positive Psychology to Realize Your Potential for Lasting Fulfillment* (New York: Free Press, 2004), 50–51.
100. Admunson, "Disability, Ideology, and Quality of Life," 104.
101. Anna Pou, "Ethical and Legal Challenges in Disaster Medicine: Are You Ready?" *Southern Medical Journal* 106, no. 1 (2013): 28–29.
102. Adrienne Asch, "Prenatal Diagnosis and Selective Abortion: A Challenge to Practice and Policy," *American Journal of Public Health* 89, no. 11 (1999): 1649–1657.

103. Ibid., 1654.
104. Susan Okie, 'Dr. Pou and the Hurricane—Implications for Patient Care during Disasters," *New England Journal of Medicine* 258, no. 1 (2008): 2.
105. Timothy Quill, "Death and Dignity—A Case of Individualized Decision Making," *New England Journal of Medicine* 324, no. 10 (1991): 691–694.
106. Okie, "Dr. Pou and the Hurricane," 4–5.
107. The classic theological text is this one: Nancy Eiesland, *The Disabled God: Toward a Liberatory Theology of Disability* (Nashville: Abingdon, 1994).
108. Pat Lyons, "Prescription for Harm: Diet Industry Influence, Public Health Policy, and the 'Obesity Epidemic,'" in *The Fat Studies Reader*, ed. Esther Rothblum and Sondra Solovay (New York: New York University Press, 2009), 75.
109. Ibid.
110. Ibid., 77.
111. Ibid.
112. Ibid., 82.
113. Gina Kolata, "Why Do Obese Patients Get Worse Care? Many Doctors Don't See Past the Fat," *New York Times*, September 25, 2016, https://www.nytimes.com/2016/09/26/health/obese-patients-health-care.html.
114. Ibid.
115. Michael Kahn, "When Battlefield Humor Backfires," *New York Times*, August 23, 2010, http://www.nytimes.com/2010/08/24/health/views/24case.html.
116. Ibid.
117. Fink, *Five Days at Memorial*, 308.
118. Ibid., 309.
119. Ibid., 243.
120. See, e.g., Megan-Jane Johnstone, *Bioethics: A Nursing Perspective*, 5th ed. (Sydney: Elsevier, 2009).
121. See Judith Wilkinson, "Moral Distress in Nursing Practice: Experience and Effect," *Nursing Forum* 23, no. 1 (1987): 16–29.
122. Harriet Washington, *Medical Apartheid: The Dark History of Medical Experimentation on Black Americans from Colonial Times to the Present* (New York: Anchor Books, 2008). For a very critical review of this book, see Ezekiel Emanuel, "Unequal Treatment," *New York Times*, February 18, 2007, http://www.nytimes.com/2007/02/18/books/review/Emanuel.t.html. This review is important for three reasons: (i) Emanuel is one of the most influential bioethicists of recent decades; (ii) he was one of the chief architects of the Affordable Care Act, otherwise known as Obamacare; and (iii) Emanuel is a proponent of "a consent substitute model" for emergency room research. Emily Largent, David Wendler, Ezekiel Emanuel, and Franklin Miller, "Is Emergency Research without Initial Consent Justified? The Consent Substitute Model," *Archives of Internal Medicine* 170, no. 8 (2010): 668–674.
123. Washington, *Medical Apartheid*, 353.

124. For a recent discussion of this issue, see Jeffrey Spike, "When Ethics Consultation and Courts Collide: A Case of Compelled Treatment of a Mature Minor," *Narrative Inquiry in Bioethics* 1, no. 2 (2011): 123–131.
125. Washington, *Medical Apartheid*, 353.
126. Ibid., 353.
127. Ibid., 358.

EPILOGUE

1. Bernadette Murphy, *Van Gogh's Ear: The True Story* (New York: Farrar, Straus and Giroux, 2016), 156.
2. Ibid., 215.
3. Ibid.
4. I would like to thank the group of pastoral theologians gathered by Robert Dykstra, who met in Philadelphia in 2018, for discussing this painting with me. Some of these observations were made by members of that group. I would like to thank in particular Jason Whitehead for his many helpful comments, especially regarding the use of light in the painting.
5. See William Meissner, "The Artist in the Hospital: The Van Gogh Case," *Bulletin of the Menninger Clinic* 58, no. 3 (1994): 283–306.
6. Brent Waters, *This Mortal Flesh: Incarnation and Bioethics* (Grand Rapids, MI: Brazos, 2009).
7. David Guinn, ed., *Handbook of Bioethics and Religion* (New York: Oxford University, 2006).
8. See, e.g., Sidney Bloch and Stephen Green, eds., *Psychiatric Ethics*, 4th ed. (New York: Oxford University Press, 2009).
9. Tom Beauchamp and James Childress, *Principles of Biomedical Ethics*, 7th ed. (New York: Oxford University Press, 2013).
10. Emmanuel Lartey, *Pastoral Theology in an Intercultural World* (Eugene, OR: Wipf and Stock, 2006), 75.
11. See Alister McGrath, *Christian Theology: An Introduction*, 3rd ed. (Oxford: Blackwell, 2001), 103.
12. Chris Adrian, "The Question," *New England Journal of Medicine* 367, no. 25 (2012): 2372.
13. Ibid., 2373.
14. Stephen Pattison, quoted in Christopher Swift, *Hospital Chaplaincy in the Twenty-First Century*, 2nd ed. (Burlington, VT: Ashgate, 2014), xiii. An important exception to the claim that "nothing has been written about chaplaincy" is this book: Wendy Cage, *Paging God: Religion in the Halls of Medicine* (Chicago: University of Chicago Press, 2012). Also see Richard Coble, *The Chaplain's Presence and Medical Power: Rethinking Loss in the Hospital System* (New York: Lexington Books, 2018).

15. See, e.g., Jann Aldredge-Clanton, *Counseling People with Cancer* (Louisville, KY: Westminster John Knox 1998).
16. In pastoral theology, two voices stand out with regard to issues of pluralism: Emmanuel Lartey and Kathleen Greider. See, e.g., Emmanuel Lartey, *In Living Color: An Intercultural Approach to Pastoral Care and Counseling* (London: Jessica Kingsley, 2003); and Kathleen Greider, "Religious Pluralism and Christian-Centrism," in *The Wiley-Blackwell Companion to Practical Theology*, ed. Bonnie Miller-McLemore (Malden, MA: Wiley Blackwell, 2012), 452–461.
17. See, e.g., Leigh Schmidt, *Restless Souls: The Making of American Spirituality* (San Francisco: Harper, 2005); and William Parsons, "On Mapping the Psychology and Religion Movement: Psychology as Religion and Modern Spirituality," *Pastoral Psychology* 59 (2010): 15–25.
18. See Thomas Cole, Nathan Carlin, and Ronald Carson, *Medical Humanities: An Introduction* (New York: Cambridge University Press, 2015).
19. See, e.g., Elizabeth Johnston Taylor, *What Do I Say? Talking with Patients about Spirituality* (Philadelphia: Templeton Foundation, 2007).
20. See, e.g., Robert Fuller, *Spiritual, but Not Religious: Understanding Unchurched America* (New York: Oxford University Press, 2001).
21. See Cole, Carlin, and Carson, *Medical Humanities*, 294–296.
22. See, e.g., Daniel Sulmasy, "A Biopsychosocial-Spiritual Model for the Care of Patients at the End of Life," *Gerontologist* 42 (2002): 24–33; and Christina Puchalski, "Spirituality and the Care of Patients at the End-of-Life: An Essential Component of Care," *OMEGA: Journal of Death and Dying* 56, no. 1 (2007-2008): 33–46.
23. Also, spiritual care is also sometimes viewed as a practice that "goes beyond an acknowledgement of religious difference (religious plurality) to creating respectful relationships for working with differences in values, beliefs, and practices (religious particularity)." See Carrie Doehring, *The Practice of Pastoral Care: A Postmodern Approach*, rev. ed. (Louisville, KY: Westminster John Knox, 2015), xxiii.
24. See Therese Jones, Delese Wear, and Lester Friedman, eds., *Health Humanities Reader* (New Brunswick, NJ: Rutgers University Press, 2014).
25. Pew Research Center, "The Changing Global Religious Landscape," April 5, 2017, http://www.pewforum.org/2017/04/05/the-changing-global-religious-landscape/.
26. See these two recent images: Jaco Hamman, "Seeing Things Differently and Not Being Looked At," *Pastoral Psychology* 58 (2009): 551–564; and Rubén Arjona, "The Librarian as an Image of Pastoral Care," *Pastoral Psychology* 65 (2016): 743–757. Also see Donald Capps, "Pastoral Images: The Good Samaritan and the Unjust Judge," *Journal of Pastoral Care and Counseling* 63, no. 1–2 (2009): 1–11.
27. See Albert Camus, *The Myth of Sisyphus, and Other Essays*, trans. Justin O'Brien (New York: Knopf, 1955).

28. William May, "Finding Common Ground in Bioethics?" in *Progress in Bioethics: Science, Policy, and Politics*, eds. Jonathan Moreno and Sam Berger (Cambridge, MA: MIT Press, 2010), 263.
29. Ibid.
30. Ibid., 263–264.
31. Ibid., 264.
32. See Donald Capps, "The Letting Loose of Hope: Where Psychology of Religion and Pastoral Care Converge," *Journal of Pastoral Care and Counseling* 51, no. 2 (1997): 139–149. Capps argued that hope is a place where psychology of religion and pastoral care converge. I suggest that moral imagination is a place where pastoral theology and bioethics converge.

BIBLIOGRAPHY

Ad Hoc Committee, Harvard Medical School. "A Definition of Irreversible Coma: Report of the Ad Hoc Committee of the Harvard Medical School to Examine the Definition of Brain Death." *JAMA* 205, no. 6 (1968): 337–340.

Adichie, Chimamanda Ngozi. "The Danger of a Single Story." TED.com, December 22, 2017. https://www.ted.com/talks/chimamanda_adichie_the_danger_of_a_single_story/transcript?language=en.

Admunson, Ron. "Disability, Ideology, and Quality of Life: A Bias in Biomedical Ethics." In *Quality of Life and Human Difference: Genetic Testing, Health Care, and Disability*, edited by David Wasserman, Jerome Bickenbach, and Robert Wachbroit, 101–124. Cambridge, UK: Cambridge University Press, 2005.

Adrian, Chris. "The Question." *New England Journal of Medicine* 367, no. 25 (2012): 2371–2373.

Akabayashi, Akira, ed. *The Future of Bioethics: International Dialogues*. New York: Oxford University Press, 2014.

Aldredge-Clanton, Jann. *Counseling People with Cancer*. Louisville, KY: Westminster John Knox, 1998.

Alexander, Shana. "They Decide Who Lives, Who Dies." *Life* 53 (1962): 102–125.

Allen, Diogenes. *Christian Belief in a Postmodern World: The Full Wealth of Conviction*. Louisville, KY: Westminster/John Knox, 1989.

Appel, Jacob. "Toward a Psychodynamic Approach to Bioethics." *American Journal of Psychoanalysis* 71, no. 1 (2011): 58–66.

Appiah, Kwame. *Cosmopolitism. Ethics in a World of Strangers*. New York: Norton, 2006.

Arjona, Rubén. "The Librarian as an Image of Pastoral Care." *Pastoral Psychology* 65 (2016): 743–757.

Arnheim, Rudolf. *Toward a Psychology of Art: Collected Essays*. Berkeley: University of California Press, 1966.

Arnheim, Rudolf. *Art and Visual Perception: A Psychology of the Creative Eye*. New version. Berkeley: University of California Press, 1974.

Arnheim, Rudolf. *New Essays on the Psychology of Art*. Berkeley: University of California Press, 1986.

Arnheim, Rudolf. *The Power of the Center: A Study of Composition in the Visual Arts*. New version. Berkeley: University of California Press, 1988.

Arnheim, Rudolf. *The Split and the Structure: Twenty-Eight Essays*. Berkeley: University of California Press, 1996.

Arnheim, Rudolf. *Visual Thinking*. Berkeley: University of California Press, 1997.

Asch, Adrienne. "Prenatal Diagnosis and Selective Abortion: A Challenge to Practice and Policy." *American Journal of Public Health* 89, no. 11 (1999): 1649–1657.

Atighetchi, Dariusch. *Islamic Bioethics: Problems and Perspectives*. Dordrecht, The Netherlands: Springer, 2007.

Baker, Robert, Arthur Caplan, Linda Emanuel, and Stephen Latham, eds. *The American Medical Ethics Revolution: How the AMA's Code of Ethics Has Transformed Physicians' Relationships to Patients, Professionals, and Society*. Baltimore: John Hopkins University Press, 1999.

Barbour, John. "The Bios of Bioethics and the Bios of Autobiography." In *Caring Well: Religion, Narrative, and Health Care Ethics*, edited by David Smith, 43–63. Louisville, KY: Westminster John Knox, 2000.

Bauby, Jean-Dominique. *The Diving Bell and the Butterfly*. New York: Vintage, 1998.

Beauchamp, Tom. "Methods and Principles in Biomedical Ethics." *Journal of Medical Ethics* 29, no. 5 (2003): 269–274.

Beauchamp, Tom. "The Philosophical Basis of Psychiatric Ethics." In *Psychiatric Ethics*, 4th ed., edited by Sidney Bloch and Stephen Green, 25–48. New York: Oxford University Press, 2009.

Beauchamp, Tom, and James Childress. *Principles of Biomedical Ethics*. 1st ed. New York: Oxford University Press, 1979.

Beauchamp, Tom, and James Childress. *Principles of Biomedical Ethics*. 7th ed. New York: Oxford University Press, 2013.

Beemsterboer, Phyllis. *Ethics and Law in Dental Hygiene*. 2nd ed. St. Louis, MO: Saunders Elsevier, 2010.

"The Belmont Report." Office for Human Research Protections. HHS.gov, last modified April 18, 1979. http://www.hhs.gov/ohrp/humansubjects/guidance/belmont.html.

"The Belmont Report 25 Years Later—Tom Beauchamp." NIH Videocasting and Podcasting. Center for Information Technology, National Institutes of Health, last modified September 22, 2004. http://videocast.nih.gov/summary.asp?Live=11549&bhcp=1.

"Bioethics." Dictionary.com, accessed on July 11, 2017. http://www.dictionary.com/browse/bioethics.

Blackhall, Leslie, Sheila Murphy, Gelya Frank, Vicki Michel, and Stanley Azen. "Ethnicity and Attitudes toward Patient Autonomy." *Journal of the American Medical Association* 274, no. 10 (1995): 820–825.

Blagg, Christopher. "The Early History of Dialysis for Chronic Renal Failure in the United States: A View from Seattle." *American Journal of Kidney Diseases* 49, no. 3 (2007): 482–496.

Bloch, Sidney, and Stephen Green, eds. *Psychiatric Ethics*. 4th ed. New York: Oxford University Press, 2009.

Blount, Brian. *Cultural Interpretation: Reorienting New Testament Criticism*. Minneapolis: Fortress, 1995.

Boisen, Anton. *The Exploration of the Inner World: A Study of Mental Disorder and Religious Experience*. Chicago: Willett, Clark, 1936.

Bowman, Kerry, and Edwin Hui. "Bioethics for Clinicians: 20. Chinese Bioethics." *CMAJ* 163, no. 11 (2000): 1481–1485.

Branch, William. "The Ethics of Caring and Medical Education." *Academic Medicine* 75, no. 2 (2000): 127–132.

Brandt, Allan. "Racism and Research: The Case of the Tuskegee Syphilis Study." In *Ethical and Regulatory Aspects of Clinical Research: Readings and Commentary*, edited by Ezekiel Emanuel, Robert Crouch, John Arras, Jonathan Moreno, and Christie Grady, 20–23. Baltimore: Johns Hopkins University Press, 2003.

Branson, Roy. "The Secularization of American Medicine." In *On Moral Medicine: Theological Perspectives in Medical Ethics*, 2nd ed., edited by Stephen Lammers and Allen Verhey 12–22. Grand Rapids, MI: Eerdmans, 1998.

Brink, Johan. "The First Human Heart and Further Advances in Cardiac Transplantation at Groote Schuur Hospital and the University of Cape Town." *Cardiovascular Journal of Africa* 20, no. 1 (2009): 31–35.

Brody, Howard. *The Healer's Power*. New Haven, CT: Yale University Press, 1992.

Brody, Baruch, and H. Tristram Engelhardt Jr. *Bioethics: Readings and Cases*. Englewood Cliffs, NJ: Prentice-Hall, 1987.

Browning, Don. *The Moral Context of Pastoral Care*. Philadelphia: Westminster, 1976.

Browning, Melissa. "Epistemological Privilege and Collaborative Research: A Reflection on Researching as an Outsider." *Practical Matters* 6 (2013): 1–16.

Brumberg, Joan Jacobs. *The Body Project: An Intimate History of American Girls*. New York: Vintage, 1998.

Buckman, Robert. *How to Break Bad News: A Guide for Health Care Professionals*. Baltimore: Johns Hopkins University Press, 1992.

Bulkeley, Kelly. *Big Dreams: The Science of Dreaming and the Origins of Religion*. New York: Oxford University Press, 2016.

Burck, J. R., and Rodney Hunter. "Pastoral Theology, Protestant." In *Dictionary of Pastoral Care and Counseling*, edited by Rodney Hunter, 867–872. Expanded ed., edited by Nancy Ramsay. Nashville: Abingdon, 2005.

Cage, Wendy. *Paging God: Religion in the Halls of Medicine*. Chicago: University of Chicago Press, 2012.

Cahill, Lisa. *Theological Bioethics: Participation, Justice, Change*. Washington, DC: Georgetown University Press, 2005.

Callahan, Daniel. *Setting Limits: Medical Goals in an Aging Society*. New York: Simon and Schuster, 1987.

Callahan, Daniel. "Religion and the Secularization of Bioethics." *Hastings Center Report* 20, no. 4 (1990): 2–4.

Callahan, Daniel. *Taming the Beloved Beast: How Medical Technology Costs Are Destroying Our Health Care System*. Princeton, NJ: Princeton University Press, 2009.

Callahan, Daniel. "Obesity: Chasing an Elusive Epidemic." *Hastings Center Report* 43, no. 1 (2013): 34–40.

Calland, Chad. "Iatrogenic Problems in End-Stage Renal Failure." *New England Journal of Medicine* 287, no. 7 (1972): 334–336.

Camus, Albert. *The Myth of Sisyphus, and Other Essays*. Translated by Justin O'Brien. New York: Knopf, 1955.

Cannon, Kelly. *Henry James and Masculinity: The Man at the Margins*. New York: St. Martin's, 1964.

Capps, Donald. *Reframing: A New Method in Pastoral Care*. Minneapolis: Fortress, 1990.

Capps, Donald. *The Depleted Self: Sin in a Narcissistic Age*. Minneapolis: Fortress, 1993.

Capps, Donald. "The Letting Loose of Hope: Where Psychology of Religion and Pastoral Care Converge." *Journal of Pastoral Care and Counseling* 51, no. 2 (1997): 139–149.

Capps, Donald. *Living Stories: Pastoral Counseling in Congregational Context*. Minneapolis: Fortress, 1998.

Capps, Donald. "The Lessons of Art Theory for Pastoral Theology." *Pastoral Psychology* 47, no. 5 (1999): 321–346.

Capps, Donald. *Giving Counsel: A Minister's Guidebook*. St. Louis, MO: Chalice, 2001.

Capps, Donald. *Laughter Ever After: Ministry of Good Humor*. St. Louis: MO: Chalice Press, 2008.

Capps, Donald. "Pastoral Images: The Good Samaritan and the Unjust Judge." *Journal of Pastoral Care and Counseling* 63, no. 1–2 (2009): 1–11.

Capps, Donald. *Erik Erikson's Verbal Portraits: Luther, Gandhi, Einstein, Jesus*. Lanham, MD: Rowman and Littlefield, 2014.

Capps, Donald. "The Minister and Mental Illness." *Pastoral Psychology* 63, no. 1 (2014): 13–22.

Capps, Donald, and Nathan Carlin. *Living in Limbo: Life in the Midst of Uncertainty*. Eugene, OR: Cascade, 2010.

Capps, Donald, and James Dittes, eds. *The Hunger of the Heart: Reflections on the* Confessions *of Augustine*. Monograph Series no. 8. West Lafayette, IN: Society for the Scientific Study of Religion, 1990.

Capps, John, and Donald Capps. *You've Got to Be Kidding! How Jokes Can Help You Think*. Oxford: Wiley-Blackwell, 2009.

Carlin, Nathan. "The Book of Job and Male Melancholia: A Bizarre Story about Hating Mother God and the Maternal Jesus, Featuring Mel Gibson." *Pastoral Psychology* 56, no. 2 (2007): 121–141.

Carlin, Nathan. "The Hospital Room as Uncanny: Psychoanalytic Observations and Recommendations for Pastors and Chaplains." *Pastoral Psychology* 58, no. 1 (2009): 27–42.

Carlin, Nathan. "The Sayings of Jesus in *Family Guy*: A Pastoral Reading of 'I Dream of Jesus.'" *Pastoral Psychology* 61, no. 4 (2012): 531–553.

Carlin, Nathan. "Bioethics and Pastoral Concern: Some Possible New Directions in Pastoral Theology." *Pastoral Psychology* 62, no. 2 (2013): 129–138.

Carlin, Nathan. "*Middlesex: A Pastoral Theological Reading*." *Pastoral Psychology* 63, no. 5–6 (2014): 561–581.

Carlin, Nathan. *Religious Mourning: Reversals and Restorations in Psychological Portraits of Religious Leaders*. Eugene, OR: Wipf and Stock, 2014.

Carlin, Nathan. "Doctors and Dr. Seuss: Restoring the Patient's Voice." *Cambridge Quarterly of Healthcare Ethics* 24, no. 1 (2015): 113–119.

Carlin, Nathan. "Medical Religion." In *Religion: Sources, Perspectives, and Methodologies*, edited by Jeffrey Kripal, 341–356. Farmington Hills, MI: Macmillan Reference USA, 2016.

Carlin, Nathan. "A Psychoanalytic Reading of *A Monster Calls*: Biblical Congruencies and Theological Implications." *Pastoral Psychology* 66, no. 6 (2017): 759–777.

Carlin, Nathan, and Donald Capps. "Consciousness, the Vegetative State, and the Intrinsic Value of Life." *Pastoral Psychology* 57, no. 5–6 (2009): 223–234.

Carlin, Nathan, and Donald Capps. *100 Years of Happiness: Insights and Findings from the Experts*. Santa Barbara, CA: Praeger, 2012.

Carlin, Nathan, Thomas Cole, and Henry Strobel. "Guidance from the Humanities for Professional Formation." In *Oxford Textbook of Spirituality in Healthcare*, edited by Mark Cobb, Christina Puchalski, and Bruce Rumbold, 443–450. Oxford: Oxford University Press, 2012.

Carson, Ronald. "Teaching Ethics in the Context of the Medical Humanities." *Journal of Medical Ethics* 20, no. 4 (1994): 237–238.

Carson, Ronald. "The Hyphenated Space: Liminality in the Doctor–Patient Relationship." In *Stories Matter: The Role of Narrative in Medical Ethics*, edited by Rita Charon and Martha Montello 171–182. New York: Routledge, 2002.

Chambers, Tod. *The Fiction of Bioethics: Cases as Literary Texts*. New York: Routledge, 1999.

Charon, Rita. *Narrative Medicine: Honoring the Stories of Illness*. Oxford: Oxford University Press, 2006.

Childress, James. "Methods in Bioethics." In *The Oxford Handbook of Bioethics*, edited by Bonnie Steinbock, 15–45. New York: Oxford University Press, 2009.

Churchill, Larry, Joseph Fanning, and David Schenck. *What Patients Teach: The Everyday Ethics of Health Care*. New York: Oxford University Press, 2013.

Clinebell, Howard. *Basic Types of Pastoral Care and Counseling: Resources for the Ministry of Healing and Growth*. Rev. ed. Nashville: Abingdon, 1984.

Coble, Richard. *The Chaplain's Presence and Medical Power: Rethinking Loss in the Hospital System*. New York: Lexington, 2018.

Cohn-Sherbok, Dan, ed. *Holocaust Theology: A Reader*. New York: New York University Press, 2002.

Cole, Thomas, Nathan Carlin, and Ronald Carson. *Medical Humanities: An Introduction*. New York: Cambridge University Press, 2015.

Collins, Patricia Hill. *Black Feminist Thought: Knowledge, Consciousness, and the Politics of* Empowerment. 2nd ed. New York: Routledge, 2000.

Cone, James. *The Cross and the Lynching Tree*. Maryknoll, NY: Orbis, 2011.

Cooper-White, Pamela. *Many Voices: Pastoral Psychotherapy in Relational and Theological Perspective*. Minneapolis: Fortress, 2007.

Cooper-White, Pamela. *Braided Selves: Collected Essays on Multiplicity, God, and Persons*. Eugene, OR: Cascade, 2011.

Couser, G. Thomas. *Signifying Bodies: Disability in Contemporary Life Writing*. Ann Arbor: University of Michigan Press, 2009.

Crawford, Hugh. "The Politics of Narrative Form." *Literature and Medicine* 11, no. 1 (1992): 147–162.

Crawford, Paul, Brian Brown, Charley Baker, Victoria Tischler, and Brian Abrams. *Health Humanities*. New York: Palgrave Macmillan, 2015.

Culbertson, Philip. *Caring for God's People: Counseling and Christian Wholeness*. Minneapolis: Fortress, 2000.

Daniels, Norman. *Just Health Care: Studies in Philosophy and Health Policy*. Cambridge, UK: Cambridge University Press, 1985.

Dasher, Jane. "Manna in the Desert: Eating Disorders and Pastoral Care." In *Through the Eyes of Women: Insights for Pastoral Care*, edited by Jeanne Stevenson Moessner, 179–191. Minneapolis: Fortress, 1996.

Davis, Dena, and Laurie Zoloth, eds. *Notes from a Narrow Ridge: Religion and Bioethics*. Hagerstown, MD: University Publishing, 1999.

DeMarinis, Valerie. *Critical Caring: A Feminist Model for Pastoral Psychology*. Louisville, KY: Westminster John Knox, 1993.

Dittes, James. "Some Accidents, Coincidents, and Intents: A Vocational Narrative." *Pastoral Psychology* 52, no. 1–2 (2003): 5–16.

Doehring, Carrie. *The Practice of Pastoral Care: A Postmodern Approach*. Rev. ed. Louisville, KY: Westminster John Knox, 2015.

Dykstra, Robert, ed. *Images of Pastoral Care: Classic Readings*. St. Louis, MO: Chalice, 2005.

Dykstra, Robert. "Unrepressing the Kingdom: Pastoral Theology as Aesthetic Imagination." *Pastoral Psychology* 61, no. 4 (2012): 391–409.

Dykstra, Robert. *Finding Ourselves Lost: Ministry in the Age of Overwhelm*. Eugene, OR: Cascade, 2018.

Dykstra, Robert, and Nathan Carlin. "At Home in the World: A Memorial Tribute to Donald Capps (1939–2015)." *Pastoral Psychology* 65, no. 5 (2016): 571–586.

Dyson, Michael Eric. *Come Hell or High Water: Hurricane Katrina and the Color of Disaster*. New York: Basic Civitas, 2005.

Edson, Margaret. *Wit: A Play*. New York: Faber and Faber, 1999.

Ehrenreich, Barbara, and Arlie Russell Hochschild, eds. *Global Woman: Nannies, Maids, and Sex Workers in the New Economy*. New York: Holt, 2002.

Eiesland, Nancy. *The Disabled God: Toward a Liberatory Theology of Disability*. Nashville: Abingdon, 1994.

Elliott, Carl. *A Philosophical Disease: Bioethics, Culture, and Identity*. London: Routledge, 1999.

Elliott, Carl. *White Coat, Black Hat: Adventures on the Dark Side of Medicine*. Boston: Beacon, 2010.

Emanuel, Ezekiel, Robert Crouch, John Arras, Jonathan Moreno, and Christine Grady, eds. *Ethical and Regulatory Aspects of Clinical Research: Readings and Commentary*. Baltimore: Johns Hopkins University Press, 2003.

Engel, George. "The Clinical Application of the Biopsychosocial Model." *American Journal of Psychiatry* 137, no. 5 (1980): 535–544.

Engelhardt, Jr., H. Tristram. *The Foundations of Bioethics*. 2nd ed. New York: Oxford University Press, 1996.

Erikson, Erik. *Insight and Responsibility: Lectures on the Ethical Implications of Psychoanalytic Insight*. New York: Norton, 1964.

Erikson, Erik. *A Way of Looking at Things: Selected Papers from 1930 to 1980*. Edited by Stephen Schlein. New York: Norton, 1987.

Evans, John. "A Sociological Account of the Growth of Principlism." *Hastings Center Report* 30, no. 5 (2000): 31–38.

Faber, Heije. *Pastoral Care in the Modern Hospital*. Translated by Hugo de Waal. Phila delphia: Westminster, 1971.

Farley, Margaret. *Just Love: A Framework for Christian Sexual Ethics*. New York: Continuum, 2006.

Feagin, Joe, and Zinobia Bennefield. "Systemic Racism and U.S. Health Care." *Social Science and Medicine* 103 (2014): 7–14.

Fenn, Richard. *Beyond Idols: The Shape of a Secular Society*. Oxford: Oxford University Press, 2001.

Fenn, Richard, and Donald Capps, eds. *On Losing the Soul: Essays in the Social Psychology of Religion*. Albany, NY: SUNY Press, 1995.

Fink, Sheri. *Five Days at Memorial: Life and Death in a Storm-Ravaged Hospital*. New York: Broadway, 2013.

Fins, Joseph. *A Palliative Ethic of Care: Clinical Wisdom at Life's End*. Sudbury, MA: Jones and Bartlett, 2006.

Flaitz, Catherine, and Nathan Carlin. "Living in Limbo: Ethics and Experience in a Conversation about Persistent Oral Lesions." *Texas Dental Journal* 128, no. 5 (2011): 427–437.

Fox, Renée, and Judith Swazey. *Observing Bioethics*. Oxford: Oxford University Press, 2008.

Frank, Arthur. *At the Will of the Body: Reflections on Illness*. Boston: Mariner, 2002.

Frankel, Richard, Timothy Quill, and Susan McDaniel, eds. *The Biopsychosocial Approach: Past, Present, Future*. Rochester, NY: University of Rochester Press, 2003.

Freud, Sigmund. *The Interpretation of Dreams*. In *The Standard Edition of the Complete Psychological Works of Sigmund Freud*, edited and translated by James Strachey. Vols. 4–5. London: Vintage, 2001. First published 1900.

Freud, Sigmund. "On Dreams." In *The Standard Edition of the Complete Psychological Works of Sigmund Freud*, edited and translated by James Strachey. Vol. 5. London: Vintage, 2001. First published 1901.

Freud, Sigmund. *Jokes and Their Relation to the Unconscious*. In *The Standard Edition of the Complete Psychological Works of Sigmund Freud*, edited and translated by James Strachey. Vol. 8. London: Vintage, 2001. First published 1905.

Freud, Sigmund. "On Humor." In *The Standard Edition of the Complete Psychological Works of Sigmund Freud*, edited and translated by James Strachey. Vol. 21. London: Vintage, 2001. First published 1927.

Fuller, Robert. *Spiritual, but Not Religious: Understanding Unchurched America*. New York: Oxford University Press, 2001.

Furman, Ben, and Ahola Tapani. *Solution Talk: Hosting Therapeutic Conversations*. New York: Norton, 1992.

Gabbard, Glen. "Boundary Violations." In *Psychiatric Ethics*, 4th ed., edited by Sidney Bloch and Stephen Green, 251–270. Oxford: Oxford University Press, 2009.

Gawande, Atul. "Whose Body Is It, Anyway? What Doctors Should Do When Patients Make Bad Decisions." *New Yorker*, October 4, 1999.

Gawande, Atul. *Complications: A Surgeon's Notes on an Imperfect Science*. New York: Picador, 2002.

Gawande, Atul. *Being Mortal: Medicine and What Matters in the End*. New York: Metropolitan Books, 2014.

Geertz, Clifford. "Thick Description: Toward an Interpretive Theory of Culture." In *Readings in the Philosophy of Social Science*, edited by Michael Martin and Lee McIntyre, 213–231. Cambridge, MA: MIT Press, 1994.

Gerkin, Charles. *An Introduction to Pastoral Care*. Nashville: Abingdon Press, 1997.

Gert, Bernard, Charles Culver, and K. Danner Clouser. *Bioethics: A Systematic Approach*. 2nd ed. New York: Oxford University Press, 2006.

Gilligan, Carol. *In a Different Voice: Psychological Theory and Women's Development*. Cambridge, MA: Harvard University Press, 1982.

Gillon, Raanan. "Ethics Needs Principles—Four Can Encompass the Rest—and Respect for Autonomy Should Be 'First among Equals.'" *Journal of Medical Ethics* 29, no. 5 (2003): 307–312.

Glass, Ira. "Tell Me I'm Fat." *This American Life*, Episode 589, June 17, 2016. http://www.thisamericanlife.org/radio-archives/episode/589/tell-me-im-fat/.

Gomes, Peter. "Introduction." In *The Courage to Be*, by Paul Tillich. 2nd ed. New Haven, CT: Yale Nota Bene, 2000.

Goodin, Robert. "No Smoking: The Ethical Issues." In *Public Health Ethics: Theory, Policy, and Practice*, edited by Ronald Bayer, Lawrence Gostin, Bruce Jennings, and Bonnie Steinbock, 117–126. Oxford and New York: Oxford University Press, 2007.

Greider, Kathleen. "Religious Pluralism and Christian-Centrism." In *The Wiley-Blackwell Companion to Practical Theology*, edited by Bonnie Miller-McLemore, 452–461. Malden, MA: Wiley Blackwell, 2012.

Groopman, Jerome. *The Anatomy of Hope: How People Prevail in the Face of Illness*. New York: Random House, 2005.

Guinn, David. ed. *Handbook of Bioethics and Religion*. Oxford: Oxford University Press, 2006.

Guinn, David. "Introduction." In *Handbook of Bioethics and Religion*, edited by David Guinn, 3–22. Oxford: Oxford University Press, 2006.

Gustafson, James. *The Contributions of Theology to Medical Ethics*. Milwaukee, WI: Marquette University Press, 1975.

Gutiérrez, Gustavo. *A Theology of Liberation: History, Politics, and Salvation*. Translated and edited by Caridad Inda and John Eagleson. Rev. ed. Maryknoll, NY: Orbis, 1988.

Habel, Norman. *The Book of Job: A Commentary*. Philadelphia: Westminster, 1985.

Hamman, Jaco. "Seeing Things Differently and Not Being Looked At." *Pastoral Psychology* 58, no. 5–6 (2009), 551–564.

Harrison, Beverly, and Shirley Cloyes. "Theology and Morality of Procreative Choice." In *Making the Connections: Essays in Feminist Social Ethics*, by Beverly Harrison and edited by Carol Robb, 115–134. Boston: Beacon, 1985.

Hawkins, Anne Hunsaker. *Reconstructing Illness: Studies in Pathography*. West Lafayette, IN: Purdue University Press, 1993.

Hawkins, Anne, and Marilyn McEntyre, eds. *Teaching Literature and Medicine*. New York: Modern Language Association, 2000.

Hiltner, Seward. *Preface to Pastoral Theology*. Nashville: Abingdon, 1958.

Holifield, E. Brooks. *A History of Pastoral Care in America: From Salvation to Self-Realization*. Eugene, OR: Wipf and Stock, 1983.

Homans, Peter, ed. *The Dialogue between Theology and Psychology*. Chicago: University of Chicago Press, 1968.

Hornblum, Allen. *Acres of Skin: Human Experiments at Holmesburg Prison*. New York: Routledge, 1999.

Horner, Jennifer. "Morality, Ethics, and Law: Introductory Concepts." *Seminars in Speech and Language* 24, no. 4 (2003): 263–274.

Hume, David. "Of Suicide." In *Essays Moral, Political, and Literary*, edited by Eugene Miller. Indianapolis, IN: Liberty Classics, 1985.

Hunter, Rodney. "A Perspectival Pastoral Theology." In *Turning Points in Pastoral Care: The Legacy of Anton Boisen and Seward Hiltner*, edited by L. Aden and J. Ellens, 53–79. Grand Rapids, MI: Baker Book House, 1990.

Hunter, Rodney, ed. *Dictionary of Pastoral Care and Counseling*. Expanded ed. Nashville: Abingdon, 2005.

Inui, Thomas. *A Flag in the Wind: Educating for Professionalism in Medicine*. Washington, DC: Association of American Medical Colleges, 2003.

Jamison, Kay. *An Unquiet Mind: Memoir of Moods and Madness*. New York: Vintage, 1996.

Johnson, Harriet McBryde. "Unspeakable Conversations." *New York Times Magazine*, February 16, 2003. http://www.nytimes.com/2003/02/16/magazine/unspeakable-conversations.html.

Johnstone, Megan-Jane. *Bioethics: A Nursing Perspective*. 5th ed. Sydney: Elsevier, 2009.

Jones, Anne Hudson. "Reading Patients—Cautions and Concerns." *Literature and Medicine* 13, no. 2 (1994): 190–200.

Jones, James. *Bad Blood: The Tuskegee Syphilis Experiment*. New exp. ed. New York: Free Press, 1993. First published 1981.

Jones, Therese, Delese Wear, and Lester Friedman, eds. *Health Humanities Reader*. New Brunswick, NJ: Rutgers University Press, 2014.

Jonsen, Albert. "Scientific Medicine and Therapeutic Choice." *New England Journal of Medicine*, 292 (1975): 126–127.

Jonsen, Albert. *A Short History of Medical Ethics*. Oxford: Oxford University Press, 2000.

Jonsen, Albert. "A History of Religion and Bioethics." In *Handbook of Bioethics and Religion*, edited by David Guinn, 23–35. Oxford: Oxford University Press, 2006.

Jonsen, Albert. "The God Squad and the Origins of Transplantation Ethics and Policy." *Journal of Law, Medicine and Ethics* 35, no. 2 (2007): 238–240.

Jonsen, Albert, Mark Siegler, and William Winslade. *Clinical Ethics: A Practical Approach to Ethical Decisions in Clinical Medicine*. New York: Macmillan, 1982.

Jonte-Pace, Diane, and William Parsons, eds. *Religion and Psychology: Mapping the Terrain*. London: Routledge, 2001.

Kaschak, Ellyn. *Engendered Lives: A New Psychology of Women's Experience*. New York: Basic Books, 1992.

Kass, Leon. *Toward a More Natural Science: Biology and Human Affairs*. New York: Free Press, 1985.

Katz, Jay. *The Silent World of Doctor and Patient*. Baltimore: Johns Hopkins University Press, 2002.

Keller, Catherine. *From a Broken Web: Sepratism, Sexism, and Self.* Boston: Beacon, 1986.

Kleinman, Arthur. *Writing at the Margin: Discourse between Anthropology and Medicine*. Berkeley: University of California Press, 1995.

Kleinman, Arthur, Veena Das, and Margaret Lock, eds. *Social Suffering*. Berkeley: University of California Press, 1997.

Kohlberg, Lawrence. *The Philosophy of Moral Development*. San Francisco: Harper and Row, 1981.

Kripal, Jeffrey. *Kali's Child: The Mystical and the Erotic in the Life and Teachings of Ramakrishna*. Chicago: University of Chicago Press, 1995.

Kripal, Jeffrey. *The Serpent's Gift: Gnostic Reflections on the Study of Religion*. Chicago: University of Chicago Press, 2007.

Kübler-Ross, Elisabeth. *On Death and Dying*. New York: Scribner, 1997.

Kuhse, Helga, and Peter Singer, eds. *A Companion to Bioethics*. 2nd ed. Malden, MA: Wiley Blackwell, 2009.

Lapsley, James. *Salvation and Health: The Interlocking Processes of Life*. Philadelphia: W estminster, 1972.

Largent, Emily, David Wendler, Ezekiel Emanuel, and Franklin Miller. "Is Emergency Research without Initial Consent Justified? The Consent Substitute Model." *Archives of Internal Medicine* 170, no. 8 (2010): 668–674.

Lartey, Emmanuel. *In Living Color: An Intercultural Approach to Pastoral Care and Counseling*. London: Kingsley, 2003.

Lartey, Emmanuel. *Pastoral Theology in an Intercultural World*. Eugene, OR: Wipf and Stock, 2006.

Lather, Patti. "Postbook: Working the Ruins of Feminist Ethnography." *Signs* 27, no. 1 (2001): 199–227.

Lebacqz, Karen. "Philosophy, Theology, and the Claims of Justice." In *Handbook of Bioethics and Religion*, edited by David Guinn, 253–263. Oxford: Oxford University Press, 2006

Lindemann, Hilde. *An Invitation to Feminist Ethics*. Boston: McGraw-Hill, 2006.

Lo, Bernard. *Resolving Ethical Dilemmas: A Guide for Clinicians*. 4th ed. Philadelphia: Wolters Kluwer Health/Lippincott Williams and Wilkins, 2009.

Lohfink, Norbert. *Option for the Poor: The Basic Principle of Liberation Theology in Light of the Bible*, 2nd ed., edited by Duane Christensen. Translated by Linda Maloney. North Richland Hills, TX: Bibal, 1995.

Lyons, Pat. "Prescription for Harm: Diet Industry Influence, Public Health Policy, and the 'Obesity Epidemic.'" In *The Fat Studies Reader*, edited by Esther Rothblum and Sondra Solovay, 75–87. New York: New York University Press, 2009.

May, William. *The Physician's Covenant: Images of the Healer in Medical Ethics*. Philad elphia: Westminster, 1983.

May, William. "Code and Covenant or Philanthropy and Contract?" In *On Moral Medicine: Theological Perspectives in Medical Ethics*, 2nd ed., edited by Stephen Lammers and Allen Verhey, 121–137. Grand Rapids, MI: Eerdmans, 1998.

May, William. "Finding Common Ground in Bioethics?" In *Progress in Bioethics: Science, Policy, and Politics*, edited by Jonathan Moreno and Sam Berger, 257–271. Cambridge, MA: MIT Press, 2010.

Mayes, Christopher. "The Harm of Bioethics: A Critique of Singer and Callahan on Obesity." *Bioethics* 29, no. 3 (2015): 217–221.

McConnell, Michael. "Equal Treatment and Religious Discrimination." In *Equal Treatment of Religion in a Pluralistic Society*, edited by Stephen Monnsma and J. Christopher Soper, 28–43. Grand Rapids, MI: Eerdmans, 1998.

McConnell, Terrance. "'She's DNR!' 'She's Research!' Conflicting Role-Related Obligations in *Wit*," in *Bioethics at the Movies*, edited by Sandra Shapshay, 186–201. Baltimore: Johns Hopkins University Press, 2009.

McEntyre, Marilyn. *Patient Poets: Illness from Inside Out*. San Francisco: University of California Medical Humanities Press, 2012.

McGrath, Alister. *Christian Theology: An Introduction*. 3rd ed. Oxford: Blackwell, 2001.

Meilaender, Gilbert. *Bioethics: A Primer for Christians*. 3rd ed. Grand Rapids, MI: Eerdmans, 2013.

Meissner, William. "The Artist in the Hospital: The Van Gogh Case." *Bulletin of the Menninger Clinic* 58, no. 3 (1994), 283–306.

Metzl, Jonathan. *The Protest Psychosis: How Schizophrenia became a Black Disease*. Boston: Beacon, 2009.

Metzl, Jonathan, and Helena Hansen. "Structural Competency: Theorizing a New Medical Engagement with Stigma and Inequality." *Social Science and Medicine* 103 (2014): 126–133.

Micheli, Jason. *Cancer Is Funny: Keeping Faith in Stage-Serious Chemo*. Minneapolis: Fortress, 2016.

Miles, Steven. *The Hippocratic Oath and the Ethics of Medicine*. New York: Oxford University Press, 2004.

Miller-McLemore, Bonnie."The Living Human Web: A Twenty-Five Year Retrospective."*Pastoral Psychology 67*, no. 3 (2018): 305–321.

Miller, Richard. "Religion, Ethics, and Clinical Immersion: An Appraisal of Three Pioneers." In *Caring Well: Religion, Narrative, and Health Care Ethics*, edited by David Smith, 17–42. Louisville, KY: Westminster John Knox, 2000.

Miller-McLemore, Bonnie. "Thinking Theologically about Modern Medicine." *Journal of Religion and Health* 30, no. 4 (1991): 287–298.

Miller-McLemore, Bonnie. "The Human Web: Reflections on the State of Pastoral Theology." *Christian Century*, April 7, 1993.

Miller-McLemore, Bonnie. "The Living Human Web: Pastoral Theology at the Turn of the Century." In *Through the Eyes of Women: Insights for Pastoral Care*, edited by Jeanne Stevenson Moessner, 9–26. Minneapolis: Fortress, 1996.

Miller-McLemore, Bonnie. "Pastoral Theology as Public Theology: Revolutions in the 'Fourth Area.'" In *Pastoral Care and Counseling: Redefining the Paradigms*, edited by Nancy Ramsay, 44–64. Nashville: Abingdon, 2004.

Miller-McLemore, Bonnie. "Revisiting the Living Human Web: Theological Education and the Role of Clinical Pastoral Education." *Journal of Pastoral Care and Counseling* 62, no. 1-2 (2008): 3–18.

Miller-McLemore, Bonnie. "The Living Human Web: A Twenty-Five Year Retrospective." *Pastoral Psychology* 67, no. 3 (2018): 305–321.

Mitchell, Juliet. *Psychoanalysis and Feminism*. New York: Basic Books, 2000.

Moessner, Jeanne Stevenson, ed. *Through the Eyes of Women: Insights for Pastoral Care*. Minneapolis: Fortress, 1996.

Moore, Zoë Bennett. *Introducing Feminist Perspectives on Pastoral Theology*. New York: Sheffield Academic Press, 2002.

Morreall, John, ed. *The Philosophy of Laughter and Humor*. Albany, NY: SUNY Press, 1987.

Morreall, John. *Comic Relief: A Comprehensive Philosophy of Humor*. Oxford: Wiley Blackwell, 2009.

Moss, Donald. "Civilization and Its Discontents: An Ongoing Update. Part 1. The Death Penalty." *Psychoanalytic Review* 88, no. 1 (2001): 87–94.

Murphy, Bernadette. *Van Gogh's Ear: The True Story*. New York: Farrar, Straus and Giroux, 2016.

Murray, Thomas. "Psychology Should Be in Dialogue with Bioethics." *Observer 15*, no. 2 (2002). http://www.psychologicalscience.org/index.php/publications/observer/2002/february-02/psychology-should-be-in-dialogue-with-bioethics.html.

Myers-Shirk, Susan. *Helping the Good Shepherd: Pastoral Counselors in a Psychotherapeutic Culture, 1925–1975*. Baltimore: Johns Hopkins University Press, 2009.

Nash, Woods. "Showing that Medical Ethics Cases Can Miss the Point: Rewriting Short Stories as Cases." *Literature and Medicine* 36, no. 1 (2018): 190–207.

Ness, Patrick. *A Monster Calls*. Ill. ed. Somerville, MA: Candlewick, 2013.

Nettle, Daniel. *Happiness: The Science behind Your Smile*. Oxford: Oxford University Press, 2009.

Nickell, Cathy Graham. *Uniting Faith, Medicine and Healthcare: A 57-Year History of the Institute for Spirituality and Health at the Texas Medical Center*. La Vergne, TN: Lighting Source, 2012.

Oden, Thomas. *Pastoral Theology: Essentials of Ministry*. New York: HarperOne, 1983.

Ofri, Danielle. *What Doctors Feel: How Emotions Affect the Practice of Medicine*. Boston: Beacon, 2013.

Okie, Susan. "Dr. Pou and the Hurricane—Implications for Patient Care during Disasters." *New England Journal of Medicine* 258, no. 1 (2008): 1–5.

Ozar, David, and David Sokol. *Dental Ethics at Chairside: Professional Principles and Practical Applications*. 2nd ed. Washington, DC: Georgetown University Press, 2002.

Pagels, Elaine. *The Origin of Satan*. New York: Random House, 1995.

Parsons, William. "On Mapping the Psychology and Religion Movement: Psychology *as* Religion and Modern Spirituality." *Pastoral Psychology* 59, no. 1 (2010), 15–25.

Patton, John. *Pastoral Care in Context: An Introduction to Pastoral Care*. Louisville, KY: Westminster John Knox, 1993.

Pembroke, Neil. *Foundations of Pastoral Counselling: Integrating Philosophy, Theology, and Psychotherapy*. Norwich, UK: SCM, 2017.

Pence, Gregory. *Classic Cases in Medical Ethics: Accounts of Cases That Have Shaped Medical Ethics, with Philosophical, Legal, and Historical Backgrounds*. 3rd ed. Boston: McGraw Hill, 2000.

Pew Research Center. "The Changing Global Religious Landscape." April 5, 2017. http://www.pewforum.org/2017/04/05/the-changing-global-religious-landscape/.

Post, Stephen. ed. *Encyclopedia of Bioethics*. 3rd ed. New York: Macmillan Reference, 2004.

Pou, Anna. "Ethical and Legal Challenges in Disaster Medicine: Are You Ready?" *Southern Medical Journal* 106, no. 1 (2013): 28–29.

Pruyser, Paul. *The Minister as Diagnostician: Personal Problems in Pastoral Perspective*. Philadelphia: Westminster, 1976.

Puchalski, Christina. "Spirituality and the Care of Patients at the End-of-Life: An Essential Component of Care." *OMEGA—Journal of Death and Dying* 56, no. 1 (2007-2008): 33–46.

Quill, Timothy. "Death and Dignity—A Case of Individualized Decision Making." *New England Journal of Medicine* 324, no. 10 (1991): 691–694.

Ramsay, Nancy. *Pastoral Diagnosis: A Resource for Ministries of Care and Counseling*. Minneapolis: Fortress, 1998.

Ramsey, Paul. *The Patient as Person: Explorations in Medical Ethics*. New Haven, CT: Yale University Press, 1970.

Rawls, John. *A Theory of Justice*. Rev. ed. Cambridge, MA: Belknap Press of Harvard University Press, 1999.

Richman, Kenneth. *Ethics and the Metaphysics of Medicine: Reflections on Health and Beneficence*. Cambridge. MA: MIT Press, 2004.

Rogers, Carl. *A Way of Being*. New York: Houghton Mifflin, 1980.

Rosen, Sidney, ed. *My Voice Will Go with You: The Psychiatric Techniques of Milton H. Erickson*. New York: Norton, 1973.

Roth, Philip. *Everyman*. Boston: Houghton Mifflin, 2006.

Rothblum, Esther, and Sondra Solovay, eds. *The Fat Studies Reader*. New York: New York University Press, 2009.

Rothman, David. *Strangers at the Bedside: A History of How Law and Bioethics Transformed Medical Decision Making*. New York: Basic Books, 1991.

Rothschild, Debra. "Partners in Treatment: Relational Psychoanalysis and Harm Reduction Therapy." *Journal of Clinical Psychology* 66, no. 2 (2010): 136–149.

Sahler, Olle, and John Carr. *The Behavioral Sciences and Health Care*. 2nd rev. ed. Cambridge, MA: Hogrefe, 2007.

Schaberg, Jane. *The Illegitimacy of Jesus: A Feminist Theological Interpretation of the Infancy Narratives*. San Francisco: Harper and Row, 1987.

Schaffer, Amanda. "The Moral Dilemmas of Doctors During Disasters." *New Yorker*, September 12, 2013.

Schmidt, Leigh. *Restless Souls: The Making of American Spirituality*. San Francisco: Harper, 2005.

Schneiderman, Lawrence, Nancy Jecker, and Albert Jonsen. "Medical Futility: Its Meaning and Ethical Implications." *Annals of Internal Medicine* 112, no. 12 (1990), 949–954.

Seligman, Martin. *Authentic Happiness: Using the New Positive Psychology to Realize Your Potential for Lasting Fulfillment*. New York: Free Press, 2004.

Selzer, Richard. "Mercy." *Iowa Review* 11, no. 2–3 (1980): 117–119.

Sharp, Melinda McGarrah. *Misunderstanding Stories: Toward a Postcolonial Pastoral Theology*. Eugene, OR: Pickwick, 2013.

Shermer, Michael. "Five Fallacies of Grief: Debunking Psychological Stages." *Scientific American*, November 1, 2008.

Shiner, Larry. "The Concept of Secularization in Empirical Research." *Journal for the Scientific Study of Religion* 6, no. 2 (1967): 207–220.

Singer, Peter. *Animal Liberation: A New Ethics for Our Treatment of Animals*. New York: Random House, 1975.

Singer, Peter. "The Singer Solution to World Poverty." *New York Times Magazine*, September 5, 1999.

Singer, Peter. *Writings on an Ethical Life*. New York: Ecco, 2000.

Singer, Peter. *One World: The Ethics of Globalization*. New Haven, CT: Yale University Press, 2002.

Singer, Peter. *Animal Liberation: The Definitive Classic of the Animal Movement*. 1st Harper Perennial ed. New York: Ecco, 2009.

Singer, Peter. *The Life You Can Save: Acting Now to End World Poverty*. New York: Random House, 2009.

Singer, Peter. *The Expanding Circle: Ethics, Evolution, and Moral Progress*. Princeton, NJ: Princeton University Press, 2011.

Singer, Peter. *Practical Ethics*. 3rd ed. New York: Cambridge University Press, 2011.

Spike, Jeffrey. "How Not to Philosophize with a Hammer: Reply to Montgomery." In *The Variables of Moral Capacity*, edited by D. C. Thomasma and D. N. Weisstub, 129–135. International Library of Ethics, Law, and the New Medicine. Vol. 21. Dordrecht, The Netherlands: Springer, 2004.

Spike, Jeffrey. "When Ethics Consultation and Courts Collide: A Case of Compelled Treatment of a Mature Minor." *Narrative Inquiry in Bioethics* 1, no. 2 (2011): 123–131.

Spike, Jeffrey, Thomas Cole, and Richard Buday. *The Brewsters: An Interactive Adventure in Ethics for the Health Professions*. 2nd ed. Houston: UTHealth, 2011.

Sugarman, Jeremy, and Daniel Sulmasy, eds. *Methods in Medical Ethics.* Washington, DC: Georgetown University Press, 2001.

Sulmasy, Daniel. "A Biopsychosocial-Spiritual Model for the Care of Patients at the End of Life." *Gerontologist 42*, suppl no. 3 (2002): 24–33.

Swift, Christopher. *Hospital Chaplaincy in the Twenty-first Century*. 2nd ed. Burlington, VT: Ashgate, 2014.

Taylor, Charles. *A Secular Age*. Cambridge, MA: Belknap Press of Harvard University Press, 2007.

Taylor, Elizabeth Johnston. *What Do I Say? Talking with Patients about Spirituality*. Philadelphia: Templeton Foundation, 2007.

Thomasma, David, and Thomasine Kushner, eds. *Birth to Death: Science and Bioethics*. New York: Cambridge University Press, 1996.

Tillich, Paul. "The Problem of Theological Method: II." *Journal of Religion* 27, no. 1 (1947): 16–26.

Tillich, Paul. *Systematic Theology*. 3 vols. Chicago: University of Chicago Press, 1973–1976.

Tillich, Paul. *Dynamics of Faith*. New York: HarperOne, 2009.

Tomiyama, A. Janet, and Traci Mann. "If Shaming Reduced Obesity, There Would Be No Fat People." *Hastings Center Report* 43, no. 3 (2013): 4–5.

Toombs, S. Kay. *The Meaning of Illness: A Phenomenological Account of the Different Perspectives of Physician and Patient*. Boston: Kluwer Academic Publishers, 1993.

Tuma, Rabiya. "Expanded-Access Programs: Little Heard Views from Industry." *Oncology Times* 30 (2008): 19, 22–23.

University of California, San Francisco. "The Kidney Project," August 7, 2017. https://pharm.ucsf.edu/kidney/need/statistics.

Wang, Lulu. "What You Don't Know." Episode 585. "In Defense of Ignorance." *This American Life*, April 22, 2016. http://www.thisamericanlife.org/radio-archives/episode/585/in-defense-of-ignorance?act=1#play.

Warren, Mary Anne. "On the Moral and Legal Status of Abortion." *Monist* 57, no. 1 (1973): 43–61.

Washington, Harriet. *Medical Apartheid: The Dark History of Medical Experimentation on Black Americans from Colonial Times to the Present*. New York: Anchor, 2008.

Waters, Brent. *This Mortal Flesh: Incarnation and Bioethics*. Grand Rapids, MI: Brazos, 2009.

Watson, James, and Francis Crick. "Molecular Structure of Nucleic Acids: A Structure for Deoxyribose Nucleic Acid." *Nature* 171, no. 4356 (1953): 737–738.

Watzlawick, Paul, John Weakland, and Richard Fisch. *Change: Principles of Problem Formation and Problem Resolution*. New York: Norton, 2011.

Wheeler, Sondra Ely. *Stewards of Life: Bioethics and Pastoral Care*. Nashville: Abingdon, 1996.

Wilkinson, Judith. "Moral Distress in Nursing Practice: Experience and Effect." *Nursing Forum* 23, no. 1 (1987): 16–29.

Wimberly, Edward. *African American Pastoral Care and Counseling: The Politics of Oppression and Empowerment*. Cleveland, OH: Pilgrim, 2006.

Wolterstorff, Nicholas. *Lament for a Son*. Grand Rapids, MI: Eerdmans, 1987.

Woodward, James, and Stephen Pattison, eds. *The Blackwell Reader in Pastoral and Practical Theology*. Malden, MA: Blackwell, 2000.

Young, Iris Marion. *Justice and the Politics of Difference*. Princeton, NJ: Princeton University Press, 1990.

Zylla, Phil. *Virtue as Consent to Being: A Pastoral-Theological Perspective on Jonathan Edwards's Construct of Virtue*. Eugene, OR: Pickwick, 2011.

Zylla, Phil. "Practices of Acceptance, Understanding and Reciprocity: Caring for Children with Disabilities and Their Families." *Pastoral Psychology* 65, no. 5 (2016): 703–715.

Zylla, Phil. "Explorations in the Aesthetic Pastoral Theology of Donald E. Capps." *Journal of Religion and Health* 57, no. 2 (2018): 538–550.

INDEX